Men's Health

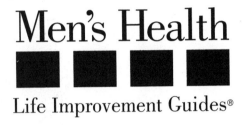

Life Improvement Guides®

Command Respect

Cultivate the Qualities
That Inspire and
Impress Others

by Perry Garfinkel, Brian Paul Kaufman,
and the Editors of **Men'sHealth**® Books

Rodale Press, Inc.
Emmaus, Pennsylvania

Copyright © 1998 by Rodale Press, Inc.

Illustrations copyright © 1997 by Alan Baseden

Men's Health Books is a trademark and *Men's Health Life Improvement Guides* is a registered trademark of Rodale Press, Inc.

Printed in the United States of America on acid-free (∞), recycled paper ♻

The Ethics Quick Test on page 61 is reprinted by permission of Texas Instruments.

The excerpt from *Making Ethical Decisions* on page 63 is by Michael Josephson. Reprinted by permission of the Josephson Institute of Ethics. Copyright © 1996.

Other titles in the *Men's Health Life Improvement Guides* series:

Fight Fat	*Powerfully Fit*	*Stronger Faster*
Food Smart	*Sex Secrets*	*Symptom Solver*
Maximum Style	*Stress Blasters*	*Vitamin Vitality*

Library of Congress Cataloging-in-Publication Data

Garfinkel, Perry.
    Command respect : cultivate the qualities that inspire and impress others / by Perry Garfinkel, Brian Paul Kaufman, and the editors of Men's Health Books.
       p.   cm. — (Men's health life improvement guides)
    Includes index.
    ISBN 0–87596–421–4 paperback
    1. Men—Conduct of life. 2. Respect. I. Kaufman, Brian, 1961– .
II. Men's Health Books. III. Title. IV. Series.
BJ1601.G37 1998
177'.1—dc21   97–33428

Distributed in the book trade by St. Martin's Press

2   4   6   8   10   9   7   5   3   1   paperback

— OUR PURPOSE —

*"We inspire and enable people to improve
their lives and the world around them."*

Command Respect Editorial Staff
Managing Editor: **Jack Croft**
Writers: **Perry Garfinkel, Brian Paul Kaufman, Alisa Bauman**
Contributing Writers: **Jennifer Barefoot, Jennifer L. Kaas, Deanna Moyer, Shea Zukowski**
Assistant Research Manager: **Jane Unger Hahn**
Lead Researcher: **Tanya H. Bartlett**
Editorial Researchers: **Elizabeth A. Brown, Deborah Pedron, Lorna S. Sapp, Carla Thomas, Teresa A. Yeykal**
Senior Copy Editor: **Amy K. Kovalski**
Copy Editor: **David R. Umla**
Series Art Directors: **Charles Beasley, Tanja L. Lipinski**
Series Designer: **John Herr**
Book Designer: **Thomas P. Aczel**
Cover Designer: **Charles Beasley**
Cover Photographer: **Mitch Mandel**
Illustrators: **Alan Baseden, J. Andrew Brubaker**
Layout Designers: **J. Andrew Brubaker, Pat Mast**
Manufacturing Coordinator: **Melinda B. Rizzo**
Office Manager: **Roberta Mulliner**
Office Staff: **Julie Kehs, Mary Lou Stephen**

Rodale Health and Fitness Books
Vice-President and Editorial Director: **Debora T. Yost**
Executive Editor: **Neil Wertheimer**
Design and Production Director: **Michael Ward**
Research Manager: **Ann Gossy Yermish**
Copy Manager: **Lisa D. Andruscavage**
Production Manager: **Robert V. Anderson, Jr.**
Studio Manager: **Leslie Keefe**
Book Manufacturing Director: **Helen Clogston**

Photo Credits
Page 146: **Courtesy of Rabbi Harold Kushner**
Page 148: **Michael Collopy**
Page 150: **Rhoda Baer**
Page 152: **Courtesy of Robyn Rodgers**
Page 154: **Andy Shivers**
Page 156: **Courtesy of Fess Parker Winery**
Back flap: **Everett Collection**

Contents

Part Five

Respect Wherever You Go

Part Six

Real-Life Scenarios

Quest for the Best

You Can Do It!

Introduction

Respectfully Yours

When I was young and foolish, I remember thinking how I never wanted to end up like my father. For some 30 years, he got up every day and went to work for the same company in a thankless, 9-to-5 job in corporate America. At the dinner table, he'd tell harrowing tales of co-workers who had been stabbed in the back, of the men who were stepped over—or on—by others as they climbed the ladder of success.

To a self-righteous and smug teenager in the 1960s, it all seemed so *pointless*. For the life of me, I couldn't figure out why anyone would put up with the daily indignities and injustices that employees were expected to swallow. But as the years passed, and I had a wife and children of my own, it gradually dawned on me.

He did it for us. For my mother, my brother, and myself.

It wasn't that my father ever viewed what he did as self-sacrifice. He did what a man was supposed to do. Work hard. Provide for his family. And pass along to his children a better life. He knew what was important in his life, and he made his decisions accordingly. Many in my generation, of course, scorned such outmoded notions. What started in the 1960s as an idealistic quest for wholeness and individuality quickly devolved into the self-absorption of the 1970s, which, in turn, mutated into the greed and conspicuous consumption of the 1980s. Today, there are men with money, power, celebrity, and all the accoutrements that come with them. They may inspire envy, curiosity, and even fear. But respect? Not hardly. It's not for sale.

We're now tasting the bitter fruit of all those years wasted on glorifying selfishness and greed. Survey after survey shows that the overwhelming majority of us believe the widespread decline in respect and accompanying increase in incivility is a major problem in society today. And part of the problem is that we don't think of respect in terms of how we live day to day. Usually, when we talk about men we respect, the conversation focuses on larger-than-life heroes, men who risked everything for their beliefs. My own list, which obviously reflects growing up in the 1960s, would include Muhammad Ali; John Lennon; Martin Luther King, Jr.; and Robert F. Kennedy. You, no doubt, have your own list.

But the men of my father's generation, the ones who fought in World War II and then built the most prosperous nation on earth, could teach us much about respect. They exemplified many of the traits and characteristics you'll read about in this book. Like integrity—having a personal moral code regarding what's right and what's wrong, and then living your life by it. Like loyalty and trustworthiness, giving your best to your employer so that you can provide the best for your family. And like altruism, giving some of your precious time to be a Boy Scout leader or to help in the local church or synagogue.

Respect, you see, isn't about some larger-than-life hero taking a courageous stand on some grand principle. It's about living every single day with integrity, honesty, confidence, and, yes, humor. Bill Maher, host of the hit ABC television show *Politically Incorrect* and a guy who knows a little about humor, once commented: "A civilization is a civilization because it is *civil*! Every little tear in the fabric of society pulls at a thread from the center until our rich tapestry looks like a doormat."

A lot of us are tired of people wiping their feet on the doormat. We're anxiously looking for ways to restore respect in the various roles that we as men are called on to play every day. *Command Respect* is our manifesto.

Jack Croft

Jack Croft
Managing Editor, *Men's Health* Books

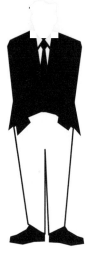

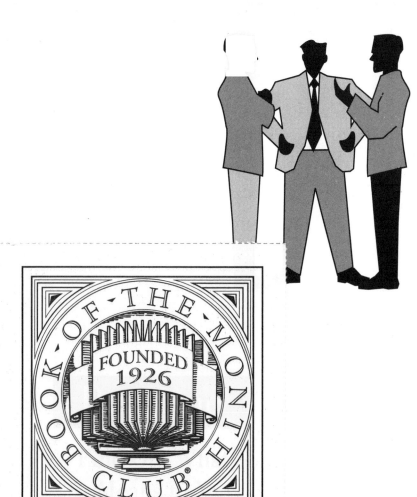

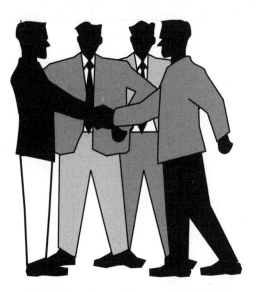

Douglas McGarvey

A Well-Respected Man

Getting What You Deserve

Item: Seven out of 10 drivers expect other drivers to treat them disrespectfully, according to a survey conducted by Bloomberg Business News. From the same survey: 80 percent of those surveyed expect disrespect from teenagers, followed by taxi drivers (62 percent), younger children (61 percent), sales clerks (58 percent), police officers (46 percent), and waiters and waitresses (35 percent).

Item: Nearly nine out of 10 Americans (88 percent) feel that incivility is a serious problem today, according to the Bozell Worldwide/*U.S. News & World Report* poll "Civility in America."

Item: A record 67 percent of Americans say that they feel alienated from people with power, money, and influence, according to the Alienation Index measured by the Harris Poll.

Item: Surveys in 1993 showed that 70 percent of students at nine state universities admitted to serious test cheating, up from 63 percent in 1963, according to Donald Mc-Cabe, Ph.D., founding president of the Center for Academic Integrity and professor of management at Rutgers University's Newark, New Jersey, campus.

Item: In a 1995 survey, 83 percent of *Men's Health* magazine readers said that men are less respected than they were 20 years earlier.

Are You Getting Any Respect?

It would not be hard to make a case for the deep and widespread erosion of respect in these times. Those factoids—added to the thousand and one real or imagined injustices of all sizes and shapes that are perpetrated on you in the course of a typical day—bring home the reality that, as comedian/nightclub owner/actor Rodney Dangerfield has so aptly (and so frequently) put it, you just don't get no respect.

Of course, no book on respect could get away without a tip of the hat to Sir Dangerfield. But not necessarily out of respect for his great talent as a comedian or thespian (please don't make us watch *Ladybugs* or *Meet Wally Sparks* to prove that). No, but because he built his career on a theme that strikes dangerously close to where every man lives.

"It's not easy bein' me," he'd complain to an audience at his Dangerfield's comedy club in Manhattan (or to anyone else who would listen), yanking at his shirt collar, his frog eyes bugging out. "Every time I get in the elevator, the operator says the same thing to me: 'Basement?'" *Rim shot!*

"That's the story of my life—no respect," he'd press on. "When I was born, the doctor told my mother, 'I did all I could...but he pulled through anyway.'" *Ba-dap bop, crash!*

What he's asking for with that familiar stage persona is sympathy. What we give him is empathy. We all can identify. We all want respect. "Men are desperate for the respect of other men," says Michael Kimmel, Ph.D., professor of sociology at the State University of New York at Stony Brook and author of *Manhood in America*. "It's such a core theme in what it means to be a man." And yet, he adds, "we don't get much of it anymore."

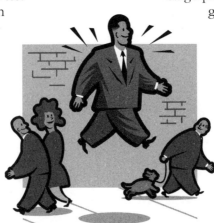

Dangerfield is a hyperbole of low self-respect, of even lower self-esteem. He portrays "a caricature of the cosmic joke we have to live with, namely, the gap between the perfection and respect we seek and the imperfection and indignity we sometimes endure," says Joel Goodman, Ed.D., director of The HUMOR Project in Saratoga Springs, New York, and co-author of *Chicken Soup for the Laughing Soul.* "The bottom line of all humor, the ability to laugh at ourselves, is a way to close that gap."

Dangerfield's caricature can be taken two ways, he adds. One is to look at his character and say, "Boy, and I thought I had it bad." Or you can live Rodney's stand-up routine, going through life complaining about how unfair it all is. That poor-me mentality can cause a downward cycle, which leads to "a negative self-fulfilling prophesy," says Dr. Goodman.

The Road to Respect

There is, however, evidence that all may not be lost after all, that respect—dare we suggest it?—may even be making a comeback.

Item: A neighborhood school in Dorchester, Massachusetts, now teaches respect to youngsters as part of its curriculum. The kids learn good manners and respectful repartee, then get to practice it in real life at an actual restaurant.

Item: At the height of the Greed Decade—that would be the 1980s—the state of California (where else?) established the Task Force to Promote Self-Esteem and Personal and Social Responsibility. The subsequent recommendations it issued on education, the family, drug and alcohol abuse, crime, violence, and poverty are "a social vaccine" helping to "unlock the secrets of healthy human development," wrote State Assemblyman John Vasconcellos of San Jose, California, who spearheaded the creation of the committee.

Item: Self-reliance and self-confidence, two important measures of self-respect, are

growing, according to the results of a survey conducted by DYG, the trend-watching organization headed by public opinion expert Daniel Yankelovich.

Item: The Borough of Raritan, New Jersey, has made illegal the use of "profane, vulgar, or indecent language by making insulting remarks or comments to others" in public places, punishable by a fine of up to $500 or 90 days in the hoosegow.

Item: Seventeen percent of students at schools without honor codes admitted to three or more serious test cheating violations, while only 7 percent reported such levels of cheating at schools with honor codes.

Item: In a series of focus groups that we hosted when we started planning the *Men's Health* Life Improvement Guides, we asked you (okay, maybe not *you* personally, but your fellow male readers) to come up with three to five adjectives that you would hope best describe you. "Respected" topped the list, hands down.

That last item is, in large part, why we wrote this book—and probably why it's in your hands right now. We men covet respect. We crave it from our fathers, our brothers, our men friends, and from the women in our lives. And while we may not agree on what it is or how to get it, we know it when we see it.

Of all the definitions of respect we heard researching this book, Dr. Kimmel offers the most bare-bones, the simplest and easiest to abide by: "It's treating people as if their integrity were equal to yours." (Our other favorite pearl of wisdom on respect comes from the mouths of babes in a children's book entitled *Learn the Value of Respect:* "You're careful with your friend's toys because you respect the property of others.")

Sometimes the easiest things to comprehend are the hardest to achieve. But by the time you get to the end of this book, you will know what to do to earn the moniker of "well-respected man." After that, it's up to you to do it.

Money and Respect

Not for Sale—At Any Price

Scholars and "Beatlemaniacs" have spent decades poring over the fab four's song lyrics, searching for hidden messages and meanings. (The walrus was Paul.) But when it comes to personal finances, the Beatles couldn't have been more on the money: "Money can't buy me love."

And neither can it buy you respect.

"A lot of people think you can purchase respect. You can't," says clinical psychologist and management consultant Steven Berglas, Ph.D., instructor of psychiatry at Harvard Medical School and author of *The Success Syndrome.* Nonetheless, Madison Avenue does nearly everything it can to encourage that idea.

"Success. It's a mind game," reads the copy on a full-page magazine ad for a Swiss watch.

"You either have it or you don't," chides a fine Scotch maker in another full-page magazine ad, apparently implying that drinking their brand will help you get "it."

"Only the best go platinum," pronounces a Platinum Guild International ad. "When it's time to measure success, nothing sets the standard like platinum."

The High Price of Success

It doesn't take a marketing wiz to know that appealing to men's competitive nature will hit a sensitive nerve. "Men constantly measure themselves against each other," says

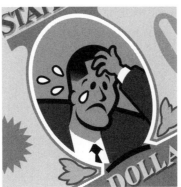

Stephen M. Pollan, a nationally known financial consultant and co-author of *Surviving the Squeeze: The Baby Boomer's Guide to Financial Well-Being in the '90s.* "In this report-card-mentality country, not surprisingly, money is the way men grade each other. We use it to decide if we have made it to the head of the class."

Those who buy in to this way of thinking—who make the attainment of money the goal and not the reward—often end up the empty-handed dunces in the corner. Or worse.

"The drive to make a lot of money generates serious mental and physical disorders," says Dr. Berglas, who works primarily with stressed-out executives in his Chestnut Hill, Massachusetts, private practice. Among the many stress-related physical disorders he sees are migraine headaches, debilitating lower-back pain, and gastrointestinal problems. On the mental side, he sees a lot of depression—both the mild variety and the severe clinical depression that leads to emotional paralysis. Others suffer from hypochondriasis, a clinical disorder or neurosis that Dr. Berglas says "derives ultimately from narcissistic preoccupation with oneself and an imbalance relating to self-esteem," traits common to men climbing the success ladder with an eerie single-mindedness.

On the personal level, Dr. Berglas also has seen men sink into distraction, isolation, and alienation, leaving irreparable cracks in their marriages and other close relationships.

To soothe the savage beasts within themselves, many men at the top often self-medicate. But it's the wrong kind: drugs and alcohol. Dr. Berglas believes a disproportionately high amount of cocaine abuse occurs among affluent men in their middle to late thirties. "These are the guys so hell-bent on money and success—

and eventually self- destruction—that they will take whatever is required to stay awake, to stay ahead," he says.

Some take drugs so that they can blame their failure on something—anything but their own ineptitude. Others take stimulants to simulate the adrenaline rush they got from competing to get where they are. Still others take depressants like booze to numb themselves from the fact that once they achieved their goal—the corner office, the lofty title, the hefty paycheck, the house in the country—the long-sought thrill was gone.

What they feel is...nothing, emptiness, nada. In their big office, with their big bucks and their big Benz, these go-getters have discovered the ugly underbelly of success.

"It's called success depression," explains Dr. Berglas, and it occurs "because success represents an ending. After spending all that time actively pursuing success, now you have nothing to look forward to. Success is a passive state."

Men used to pushing buttons, metaphorically speaking, now have nothing to do but count their money and read their press clippings. It's easy for men who've been taught that their male identities come from doing—not being—to lose a sense of self-worth and sink into a funk. Many of the so-called white-collar crimes are committed not by men desperate to succeed, Dr. Berglas points out, but by men bored with their status quo. Like upscale suburban teenagers who go on theft sprees, these men try to regenerate interest in their jobs by outwitting the establishment.

"Men like this talk to me about feeling no satisfaction or self-esteem from their work, about lacking self-respect, about viewing themselves as something contemptible," Dr. Berglas says.

Be Like Mike

Chicago Bulls professional basketball star Michael Jordan is a perfect example of a man who discovered that all the success and money in the world may not be enough. In 1993, at the pinnacle of his athletic career—three NBA championships and the leading scorer for more years in a row than any other player—he quit. At the age of 31, he felt the thrill was gone and that he couldn't possibly earn any more respect. "Michael always said that when basketball stopped being fun, he was going to walk away," coach Phil Jackson wrote in his book *Sacred Hoops*.

Jordan decided to start over, this time in baseball. He took the Horatio Alger route, attempting to rise from the bottom of the minor leagues. Sports fans know he failed. But did he? In 1995, he returned to basketball, and a year later the Bulls won their fourth championship. He was back on top of the league, and all was right with the world (at least the basketball world) again. Those who watched the end of that last championship game on TV saw the cameras follow Jordan into the locker room, where he bawled like a baby, his arms wrapped around the ball. No one could argue that he had regained a love of the game—and, in the process, no small degree of respect both for himself and from us.

"It was climbing the ladder again that made him so happy," says Harvard Medical School's Dr. Steven Berglas, author of *The Success Syndrome*. "That's the key to rebuilding self-respect."

Rags to Riches

So if the pot of gold at the end of the rainbow is not what earns respect, what does? It's the long climb up the steep ladder—and the further the climb, the more we respect it.

"We respect people who have distanced themselves from their origins," Dr. Berglas says. We are always moved and motivated by the rags-to-riches story of the man who started with squat and built it into a fortune, the immigrant who arrived on the ship with $10 in his pocket and now owns the shipping line. We admire and respect the man who fought against all odds to win the race, the contract, the girl. We want to be known as the guy who made it the hard way, who charted the new road across the top of the rocky mountain in a four-wheel drive rather than take the paved road around it in a four-door, air-conditioned sedan.

"Anything related to rugged individualism is part of the image of masculinity we hold sacred," says Dr. Michael Kimmel of the State University of New York at Stony Brook. "People have always derived more self-esteem from having a vision and actualizing it than getting a paycheck and living off it."

That's surely why Abraham Lincoln perennially tops polls as America's greatest president. As much as his stand against slavery and his handling of the Civil War, we respect his rise from the boy who taught himself by candlelight in the backwoods Kentucky log cabin where he was born to 16th president of the United States.

So if money isn't earning you respect or a sense of satisfaction and fulfillment, Dr. Berglas suggests that you re-examine your priorities. Look backward, not forward. Pull out your old high school yearbook and remind yourself of what you used to do for fun. "Make the things that you were once passionate about important in your life again," Dr. Berglas says. "Do something that you want to wake up to every day."

The concept of being trapped in what corporate America calls golden handcuffs—stuck in a job you hate that pays too well to quit—isn't about being addicted to the paycheck. It's about being thwarted from following your dream. Follow your dream and instead of following the money, the money will follow you.

The Pursuit of Happiness

Now that you've given up striving to gain respect by amassing tons of money, you may want to know how to stock up on that ever-elusive commodity that will really earn you big points among your friends. It's right there in the Declaration of Independence. The pursuit of happiness is one of our "unalienable rights." Nonetheless, the attainment of it seems to be slipping away. Only 32 percent of those surveyed in the 1996 University of Chicago's National Opinion Research Center's General Social Survey (financed by the federal government) said that they were very happy.

For those who do find it, there's a non-financial payoff to being happy. "Happy people tend to be more creative, more trusting, more loving, more decisive, and—in the well-replicated so-called feel good, do good phenomenon—more altruistic," says David Myers, Ph.D., professor of psychology at Hope College in Holland, Michigan, and author of *The Pursuit of Happiness*. All these are highly respectable characteristics. Dr. Myers outlines the following strategies for not just pursuing but actually attaining true happiness.

Keep your eye on the right prize. Repeat this mantra: "Money doesn't buy happiness." In fact, wealth is like health. "Its utter absence breeds misery, but having it (or anything else we long for) doesn't guarantee happiness," says Dr. Myers.

Savor the moment. Happiness, said Benjamin Franklin, "is produced not so much by great pieces of good fortune that seldom happen as by little advantages that occur every day." In other words, slow down and smell the cappuccino.

Master time. Happy people feel in control of their lives. They set daily achievable goals and meet them. Maybe you won't get to everything on your daily to-do list, but after a year you'll be impressed at how much you've accomplished. And be happy for that.

Get in character. We can act ourselves into any frame of mind. When smiling, people feel better; when they scowl, the whole world scowls back. So, though it may sound like a cliché, "put on a happy face," Dr. Myers advises. Going through the motions of positive feeling can trigger those precise results.

Get engaged. To your work or play, that is. "Happy people are often in a zone called flow—absorbed in a task that challenges them without over-whelming them," says Dr. Myers. View what you do as a challenge, not a chore. And that applies whether it's your work or your workout.

Move. Aerobic exercise not only promotes health and energy but also acts as a mild antidote for depression and anxiety. Sound minds reside in sound bodies.

Sleep it off. The growing national sleep debt is costing Americans a fair share of happiness. Lack of sleep causes fatigue, diminished alertness, and gloomy moods. Short of getting some actual Zzzs, Dr. Myers recommends a day of R.E.S.T.: Restricted Environmental Stimulation Therapy. In other words, hang the "Gone fishin'" sign on your psychic office door and take a day off for yourself.

Stay close. "There are few better remedies for unhappiness than an intimate friendship with someone who cares deeply about you," Dr. Myers says. Confiding is good for body and soul. Don't take partners for granted. Allow them to really get to know you, rather than keeping them at arm's length.

Nourish your soul. Dr. Myers points to a number of studies that show that actively religious people are happier. They cope better with crisis. Faith provides a support community, a sense of life's meaning, feelings of ultimate acceptance, something beyond oneself to focus on, and a timeless perspective on life's woes.

Money Isn't Everything

Cuba Gooding, Jr., won an Academy Award in 1997 for making a mantra of the line, "Show me the money" in the film *Jerry Maguire*. Gooding's character, a football player, got his sports agent Jerry Maguire, played by Tom Cruise, to chant, then maniacally shout the line with him into the phone. It's the ultimate humiliation Maguire suffers to save his career from going down the toilet. The agent redeems his self-esteem and earns our respect by making a big comeback and getting his client to play for the love of the game, and *not* for the money.

The film resonates with men because that's the direction many of us are already moving in, according to a survey conducted by DYG, the social trend–analyzing firm chaired by public opinion expert Daniel Yankelovich. The results show that men are developing their own parameters of respect. For example:

- We're defining success on our terms. Sixty-four percent of men embraced the idea that "my sense of success comes from the way I feel about myself, not from what others think."
- We're de-emphasizing success based on material possessions. We're dumping the yardstick of bigger, better, and more toys—cars, stereos, you name it—as a measure of success. Fifty-eight percent support the idea that "we place too much emphasis on the reward you get from the things one can buy."
- Money isn't enough. Men feel that they should be getting more than just money from their work. Fifty-six percent of those surveyed believe that "no matter how much a job pays, it's no good if it doesn't provide personal gratification."

Power and Respect

Defining It on Your Own Terms

You can talk about...

...the power of a Porsche engine; the power of a Ken Griffey, Jr., swing; the power of the atomic bomb; the power of a bank president; the power of the President of the United States; the power of knowledge; the power of the press; the power of attorney; the power to create and the power to destroy; the power of love; the power of prayer; the power to reason, to know right from wrong, to hold on to what's important and to let go of what's not; the power to take charge of one's life, to turn boyhood dreams into the fulfillment of manhood.

Power is the buzzword of our times: power ties, power lunches, power brokers, power mongers, power trippers, power chords, power plays, superpowers. And, for better or worse, it is the yardstick by which we measure our manhood. Either you're on the power bus (probably driving it) or you're not (probably being flattened into roadkill by it). Power can motivate us to greatness. Or it can drive us into a downward spiral of deception and corruption.

For many of us, it's the Holy Grail of Respect. And like the knights of King Arthur's court, we're chasing after an illusion. "I'm not so sure power earns men's respect," says Dr. Michael Kimmel of the State University of New York at Stony Brook. "It may earn men's fear. It may earn men's deference."

But respect? That's another matter.

Power Struggle

"Of all the aspects of our lives, power remains one of the least understood and most important—especially for our generation." Though Alvin Toffler, author of *Future Shock* and *The Third Wave*, wrote those words in *Powershift* in 1990, they are as relevant today, and we're quite sure will continue to be so well into the next millennium.

So what is power? It always comes down to control, over your own life and actions, or over the lives and actions of others. The issue of whether men exercise control is highly charged and based on your perspective. Listen as two of the leading experts on men's issues weigh in on the subject, drawing polar opposite conclusions.

"If power means having control over one's life, then men have little or no power," proclaims psychologist Warren Farrell, Ph.D., author of *The Liberated Man*, *Why Men Are the Way They Are*, and *The Myth of Male Power*. "What we've learned to call power is powerlessness. For example, the obligation to earn money that someone else spends while we die sooner sounds more like enslavement to me than power."

Dr. Kimmel could not disagree more. Commenting on Dr. Farrell's point, he says, "That's a *feeling*, and I can't argue with a feeling. Sure, guys say, 'I have no power. My wife bosses me around. My kids boss me around. My boss bosses me around.' But as a sociologist, I must note those feelings don't correspond with empirical reality. On a societal level, we men have privileges that come to us solely by virtue of being men."

No matter how you define it or whether you think you have it, chances are that you want it, says Andrew Kimbrell, director of the International Center for Technology Assessment in Washington, D.C., co-founder

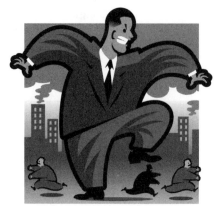

of The Men's Health Network, and author of *The Masculine Mystique: The Politics of Masculinity.* "The drive for dominance and power is, of course, a fundamental aspect of the masculine mystique," he writes. "It is the ticket to manhood, freedom, and respect." Or so we have been led to believe.

Men in Power

The problem is that power often comes at the expense of others' respect, at the expense of one's own health, at the expense of one's relationships, and—ultimately—at the expense of one's own self-respect.

It's not that power and respect are mutually exclusive. But it has been amply demonstrated that one does not necessarily lead to the other.

Why? Because the things men sometimes have to do to rise to positions of power do not make for a pretty picture, certainly not a respectable picture, says F. G. Bailey, Ph.D., emeritus professor of anthropology at the University of California, San Diego, and author of several books, including *Humbuggery and Manipulation: The Art of Leadership* and *The Prevalence of Deceit.*

"A leader is not necessarily someone who does great things," Dr. Bailey says. "It's someone who commands followers—makes them do what he (or she) wants. He can do this in a variety of ways: intimidate them, bribe them, trick them, brainwash them into sacrificing themselves for a cause in which he himself may or may not believe. It follows that a successful leader is (a) not bound by the conventions of his own society, and (b) perfectly willing to use other people as instruments rather than as human beings entitled to their own dignity." In

Atten-hut!

If the thought of a Marine drill instructor makes you cower in your boots, then you may just soil your Skivvies when you encounter Gunnery Sergeant David Camacho. He trains drill instructors at the Marine Corps Recruit Depot on Parris Island, South Carolina.

This man commands respect—literally. Here he shares some of the wisdom that helped make the Marines one of the world's most highly respected combat forces.

Discipline only when necessary. "It's easy to be hard—it's hard to be smart," says Camacho. "Anybody can discipline a recruit. The magic is for them to know how and why they are being disciplined." A recruit who doesn't know why he's being disciplined loses respect for the drill instructor. He assumes that his instructor is exercising his power of authority because he can—and for no other reason. We've all worked for people like that—and lost respect for them for the same reason.

Be positive. Even when your recruits look like they're going to be a serious project, you should "believe in them because if you don't, how can you expect others to?" asks Camacho. "If you think recruits are losers, that's the way they'll turn out because that's the subliminal thought you're sending." The Marine way: Simply replace negative thoughts with positive ones. The job you can't finish in time? Just remind yourself that you've beaten deadlines before—you'll do it again.

Speak in a "command voice." Don't scream from your throat; that comes out whiny and nasal and you'll be hoarse before boot camp is over. "Bring it up from the gut," says Camacho, meaning your diaphragm. "First get people's attention with a preparatory command. The next words out of your mouth should be an imperative: Execute this order."

his view, a man in power is not big on the Golden Rule.

Neither is this a person who will attract a trusting circle of friends. "Just as he is insensitive to the needs and feelings of others, a leader also has a perfectly irrational confidence in himself, an ability to close off self-criticism, and the capacity to disregard reality and believe in the inevitability of his ultimate victory," adds Dr. Bailey. It will indeed be lonely at the top for this guy.

Can leaders have the respect of their own community? "Yes," says Dr. Bailey, "to the extent that they can conceal all those features that I have just listed and present themselves as honest, sincere, considerate, rational, and intelligent."

By Dr. Farrell's accounting, men pay a high price for power. The power motive has put us in a deep hole—almost literally, he says. He attributes the fact that women live, on average, about seven years longer than men to the additional stress and strain men experience being the breadwinner in most families in industrialized societies.

In an effort to provide for those they love, many men fall into the trap of working long hours to earn more money. As a result, they spend increasingly less time with their loved ones—an outcome that Dr. Farrell calls the male tragedy. By being absent from our children's lives in pursuit of the power carrot, we are a poor role model. By being absent from our wives' and lovers' lives or exhausted when we do finally come home after a long day, they lose our presence and we lose their respect.

The isolation of being in power—call it the lonely-at-the-top syndrome—may cost lives. Research shows that loneliness is a strong predictor of heart disease.

Claims to Fame

Don't confuse fame with accomplishment, advises Joshua Gamson, Ph.D., assistant professor of sociology at Yale University and author of *Claims to Fame: Celebrity in Contemporary America*. And don't misinterpret fame as the way our culture bestows respect. It isn't.

It used to be that you had to *do* something to earn fame. Now it seems the rules of the fame game have changed.

Fame is "the ability to stand out from the crowd," according to Dr. Gamson's definition. "In a culture this mass and massive, standing out is an achievement in itself," he notes. But just because people are famous doesn't mean they did something worthy of respect. "Visibility itself has come to be something our culture respects, rather than the things one does to earn that visibility," he says.

A self-confessed reader of *People* magazine and watcher of *Entertainment Tonight*, Dr. Gamson says the famous people who earn his respect "show some signs of intelligence, have a broader view of what they're doing, an ability to express themselves, and quirkiness (that tops my list). They're people who take genuine risks, who have some belief system that goes beyond commerce."

The New Power Generation

Today, with the rampant takeover of so many aspects of our lives—from multinational corporations to unwanted Muzak in elevators—how does a man gain control in his own life? He starts by taking responsibility for his life and setting his own standards of success. This is illustrated by the results of a survey of men conducted jointly by *Men's Health* magazine and public opinion expert Daniel Yankelovich's DYG, a social trend–watching organization. Called ManScan: The New Status, it identifies

Andy Warhol, that pop culture icon of the 1960s, once said, "In the future, everybody will be world-famous for 15 minutes." So have you had yours? We thought not. The problem must be in your marketing strategy. With Dr. Gamson's consultation (and tongue planted firmly in cheek), we've drafted these do-it-yourself instructions for getting famous.

1. Rescue a small child from danger, like the bottom of a well.
2. Get a publicist.
3. Write a book.
4. Commit a grandiose act of altruism.
5. Get a manager.
6. Write a sequel to your first book.
7. Sleep with someone truly famous.
8. Get a Hollywood agent.
9. Write a screenplay based on your life.
10. Become a spokesman for a weight-loss program or an exercise machine.
11. Produce a video.
12. Get a bodyguard.
13. Appear in a public place in woman's attire.
14. Get a shrink.
15. Get a life!

the values men hold dearest. Consider it a snapshot of men as we march en masse into the next millennium. The common theme? "Taking control of their own lives and their own idea of personal success," report the researchers, who add that men are showing "an almost-contrarian optimism built on self-reliance."

- There's confidence in the face of confusion. Despite the vagaries of life—corporate downsizing, crime, divorce, to name a few of the more prickly thorns these days—57 percent of the men surveyed agreed with this statement: "I feel better about myself than I ever have."
- Self-reliance fuels optimism. Eighty-two percent of respondents agreed with the statement, "I feel that by being smart about my choices, I can create a good life."
- Fitness matters. Being fit is one of the personal choices that men feel makes a difference. Seventy-seven percent agreed with the comment, "Being physically fit gives me more confidence."
- Life is getting better. Despite the fact that so much of life is up for grabs, men say they feel more in control than ever. Sixty-six percent agreed with the following: "I have better control over the direction of my life compared to five years ago."
- Like father, like son. Men are split evenly on how their lives compare with their fathers'. Fifty-one percent agreed with the statement, "I have better control over the direction of my life than my father did."

But who needs surveys and studies to substantiate all this? You can read the same message in the things we buy. "We sometimes wear power as if it were a fashion accessory," Dr. Kimmel says. Men demonstrate their desire to control their lives and tame their environment by buying four-wheel-drive jeeps to drive through city streets, by wearing hiking boots to walk around the mall, or dousing themselves in colognes with names like Safari. These consumer behaviors all shout, "I, Tarzan, king of my jungle." Just be careful, warns Dr. Kimmel, that you're not substituting these material acquisitions for the real thing. Taken to extremes, "this is impotence masquerading as power," he says.

Being a Man

The New Masculinity

It used to be so easy to be a man.

There was huntin'. *Grrrrrr.* Gatherin'. *Grunt.* Eatin'. *Crunch.* Sleepin'. *Zzz.* And, er, procreatin'. Mmmmmmmmm.

That was a day in the life of your average well-respected Caveman About Town. And, as long as you lived to talk about your many conquests over roast woolly mammoth around the campfire that evening, you got a lot of respect for your efforts.

Then it got all mucked up. Governments. Religions. Wars. The Industrial Revolution. The Sexual Revolution. The Women's Movement. The Men's Movement. Macho Man. Sensitive Man. Wild Man. And Macho Man Redux, also known as the Alpha Male.

Respect? Man, you felt lucky if someone returned your phone call.

As if this wasn't confusing enough, somebody kept changing the rules of respect. Heck, that same somebody (we now suspect there was more than one "somebody") threw out the whole rule book on what it meant to be a man. The very basics of male identity—assumptions we considered as fundamental to our survival as a hunk of steak and crispy french fries—were being questioned. Some even went so far as to question whether those steaks and fries were essential for our survival.

A Man's Man

All we really wanted was a little respect from our fellow hunters and gatherers, says Dr. Michael Kimmel of the State University of New York at Stony Brook.

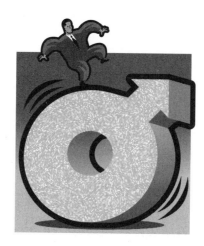

"What we really want and need from our fathers, our teachers, our men friends is that they see us as manly—as a man's man, as a man among men," Dr. Kimmel says. "That's very, very important to us. I think it is the crucial theme in masculinity."

Agreed. But with all due respect, Doc, what precisely is manly? What is a man's man? What's masculinity? And how do they all relate to respect?

To all of which Dr. Kimmel unequivocally responds: It depends.

"Manhood means different things at different times to different people," Dr. Kimmel says. "Manhood is neither static nor timeless." For American men, he says, "it depends heavily on one's class, race, ethnicity, age, sexuality, and geographic region you grew up in." It is, he goes on, created in and by our culture. What is consistent, he suggests, is that we seem to ask the hard questions and probe for what it truly means to be a man during moments of crisis and transition—whether personally or as a society—"when old definitions no longer work and the new definitions are yet to be firmly established."

You're reading this book at just such a moment. At least from a societal perspective. We suspect you've been grappling with the issue on a personal level as well. But you're not alone.

In the 1995 Virginia Slims Opinion Poll conducted by Roper Starch Worldwide, 62 percent of the men surveyed said "more and more men are questioning the 'macho' role," and 80 percent said "people admire men who show a more sensitive side."

A Time of Transition

So where does that leave men today? "It's hard for men to feel respect when the rules of masculinity keep changing," says Ronald F. Levant, Ed.D., associate clinical professor of psychology in the department of psychiatry at Harvard Medical

School and author of *Masculinity Reconstructed, Between Father and Child*, and other books about men. Working on the old premise, he says, "the standards of masculinity were: compete; achieve; be stoic; don't express vulnerabilities; be dependable, strong, and self-reliant; be cool-headed, logical, and reasonable; be decisive.

"It's complicated now because the old rules don't hold sway and the new rules haven't been agreed on," he adds. "We assumed if we followed the rules, we'd get respect. But it's a whole new ball game."

In a study he conducted, Dr. Levant found responses "strikingly different from the conventional wisdom about the beliefs men hold" in seven key categories. Here's what he found.

- Men have loosened up a lot on what behavior they consider appropriate for men only and women only. Men now believe it's okay for males to enjoy needlecraft and wear bracelets without threatening their masculinity.
- Men are rejecting the old stereotype of the strong, silent type. Those in the study said showing emotions such as fear, worry, and love for their fathers was perfectly acceptable.
- Men are no longer expected to always be "the stud," eager whenever an opportunity for sex comes up. They were more inclined to connect sex with intimacy.
- Men are beginning to realize that achievement isn't the only thing that matters, and they are more willing to share power and status with women.
- Men are still committed to the idea that masculinity and self-reliance are closely related, but now it's okay, for example, to ask for help in changing a tire. They disagreed with the statement, "A man should never doubt his judgment."

The Whole Ball of Wax

Okay, it's only a wax museum, but it's the most famous wax museum in the world: Madame Tussaud's Waxworks Museum in London. Since 1970, visitors to the museum have been asked to name the people past or present whom they considered the most heroic. They named only two women in all those years: Mother Teresa and Joan of Arc. Here's a rundown (in the order of their popularity) of how the list has shaped up every five years.

- **1973:** Jesus, Winston Churchill, John F. Kennedy, Moshe Dayan
- **1978:** Winston Churchill, Superman, Muhammad Ali, Horatio Nelson, John F. Kennedy
- **1983:** Superman, Joan of Arc, Martin Luther King, Jr., Mother Teresa, Elvis Presley
- **1988:** Superman, John Wayne, Winston Churchill, Clint Eastwood, Sylvester Stallone
- **1993:** Harrison Ford, Arnold Schwarzenegger, Superman, Sylvester Stallone, Mahatma Gandhi

---

- Men still value the traits of strength, courage, and aggression, but they are now discriminating between healthy and unhealthy forms of aggression.
- There are signs that men have "worked free enough of homophobia" to disagree fairly strongly with the statement that a man should end a friendship with another man if he finds out the other man is a homosexual.

Acting Out

Masculinity is something that "we act out in front of each other," suggests Dr. Kimmel. In other words, we are each other's mirrors. We can define masculinity—and we define respect—by the friends we keep.

If that is the case, then the results of a survey by DYG, a group that tracks social trends, should shed some light on the subject. These are the qualities men say they admire in another man (and, in parentheses, the percentage who named that attribute). We admire a man who is dependable (88 percent), honest (88), authentic and not phony (79), smart (65), will roll up his sleeves (86), balances work and leisure (65), has good relationships with family and friends (83), has a sense of humor (81), and is a regular guy (69).

All of this suggests that men are now doing a lot more introspective thinking about a subject near and dear to their hearts: themselves. And that has led to redefining what we respect in each other. Since those prehistoric days of clubs and loincloths, men have defined themselves by external achievements, points out Tony Trigilio, Ph.D., lecturer in English at Northeastern University in Boston and area chair in masculinities for the American Culture Association based at Bowling Green State University in Ohio. Now, it's no longer enough to know *what* you've done. We also want to know *why* you did it. We want to understand what makes you tick, what motivates you as a man.

"Men are desperate for the respect of other men," Dr. Kimmel says. "Ironically, though, we don't seem to be able to get much of it." That has as much to do with our diminishing respect for social institutions as it does for individuals. We used to draw our sense of self from family, from schools, and from our religious affiliation. Now, families struggle to stay together; schools often seem to be fighting to remain safe environments first and educational centers second; and the influence of religion has waned in the lives of many, Dr. Kimmel says.

The number of adult Americans who said they attended a church or synagogue once

The Crying Game

One of the reasons that women are more likely to shed tears than men has nothing to do with emotions. Biologically, women have higher levels of the hormone prolactin, which helps in the production of milk. Crying is one way to release excess quantities of prolactin.

About 80 percent of men report that they never—or hardly ever—cry, while the same percentage of women say they cry on a regular basis, according to Jeffrey Kottler, Ph.D., professor of counseling and educational psychology at Texas Tech University in Lubbock, Texas, and author of *The Language of Tears*.

Men cry less often, shed fewer tears, and make less noise when they do, Dr. Kottler says. According to one study, men are eight times less likely than women to cry when they are yelled at and nine times less likely to cry at sentimental gatherings. We're also less inclined to use tears manipulatively.

"In interviews, men told me poignant stories of how they were shamed by their fathers or coaches to stop crying somewhere around age 13," Dr. Kottler says. He discovered that such experiences aren't unique to American

a week or more fell from 51 percent in 1986 to 43 percent in 1994, according to a survey conducted by Louis Harris and Associates. On the other hand, the number of adults who said they went to movies at least once a month has increased from 23 percent to 31 percent from 1990 to 1995, according to the International Motion Picture Almanac.

Reel Respect

Who were the men who most influenced you when you were coming of age? Culturally males. In Africa, for example, young men who cry when they go through public ritual circumcision won't marry well and won't obtain a position of status in their communities.

"Men cry in response to feelings that are part of their core identity," Dr. Kottler says. "That identity is framed in the roles of provider, protector, warrior, athlete, husband, father, and team player. Male tears are more inclined to express experiences of pride, bravery, loyalty, victory, and defeat."

Traditionally, tears are a visible sign of emotional instability and vulnerability, not attributes typically admired in men. But "the rules are changing now for men," says Dr. Kottler.

Starting with Ronald Reagan, whom he calls a "free crier," crying seems to be presidential style. George Bush cried in public. One researcher estimated Bill Clinton cried at least three dozen times in his first term alone—and every time, his approval ratings went up afterward.

General Norman Schwarzkopf, of Desert Storm fame, said, "I don't think I would like a man who is incapable of enough emotion to get tears in his eyes."

So let those ducts go and those tears flow. They may help you win your next election.

and historically, they were movie stars, celluloid icons of masculinity, according to Joan Mellen, Ph.D., professor of English at Temple University in Philadelphia and author of *Big Bad Wolves: Masculinity in the American Film.*

Pick your era. From the early days of film, there was Tom Mix, Gene Autry, Errol Flynn, Gary Cooper, John Wayne. Or were you into James Dean or Marlon Brando in the 1950s? Or later still, Sylvester Stallone, Arnold Schwarzenegger, or Tom Cruise. Or the man whose career seemed to transcend and overshadow them all: Clint Eastwood.

A lot of men came out of movie theaters, testosterone bubbling over their popcorn, thinking that these were the heroes they most wanted to emulate. But were the traits they projected all that admirable? "With the perspective of hindsight, not at all," says Dr. Mellen. Through these men, we learned that to be respected, we must always succeed alone, we must get the "enemy" before he gets us, and we must be a man of few words.

The male movie hero "was judged by how silently he could endure the rigors of his life," Dr. Mellen continues. "His solace had to come not from what were considered weak-minded confessions of uncertainty, regret, or fear, but from inner strength, self-confidence, and pride in tasks well-done. To talk too much would violate this code and demean his mission. The more silent the hero, the greater his nobility and the more, illogically, we were urged to trust him."

Meanwhile, Dr. Mellen points out another negative by-product of substituting screen heroes for real-life men worthy of our respect. Film, and especially American film, has given us bigger-than-life male characters who loom over us on the silver screen, casting gray shadows of self-doubt on us by their very magnitude. "Hollywood has known well that men cannot live by its models of masculinity," says Dr. Mellen. Such heroic images—capable of feats of power and control inaccessible to mere mortals—have afforded men vicarious release while rendering them small and timid by comparison. "When men left the theater, catharsis behind them," she says, "they were left with nothing so much as an overwhelming sense of their own inadequacy. In seeming to entertain us, movies in a very real sense have exacerbated our pain."

The Well-Spoken Man

Having Your Way with Words

It's not always what you say but how you say it that shows someone respect. Sure, "please" and "thank you" pave the respect way. "Sir" or "ma'am" also bestow respect. Not interrupting, not using profanity, not barking out orders—these are the givens of respectful conversation.

"But it's what we say between the words that tells a person that you respect him or her and that earns their respect," says Suzette Haden Elgin, Ph.D, director of the Ozark Center for Language Studies in Huntsville, Arkansas, and author of *How to Disagree without Being Disagreeable.* With 90 percent of the emotional information we send contained in nonverbal communication, she says, that puts a big weight on body language and intonation.

Of course, it wouldn't hurt to take a course entitled "30 Days to a More Powerful Vocabulary." The well-spoken man often knows how to turn a phrase or throw in the occasional impressive $10 word. That always lends a little *élan.* But trying to impress people with highfalutin multisyllabic words can easily become transparent when someone asks you to define *élan*—and you have no idea what it means.

Speaking of Respect...

Since everyone defines respect by their own standards, Dr. Elgin advises using the simplest rules to cover the broadest range of possibilities when trying to maintain respectful communications.

Be formal first. "Always begin with the most formal form of address," suggests Dr. Elgin. Mr., Mrs., Ms.: That's a safe start. If you try to decide beforehand who deserves more or less respect—older men, younger men, older women, younger women, doctors, lawyers, Indian chiefs—you will probably inadvertently step on someone's toes. Address John Q. Public as Mr. Public. He may well tell you, "Oh, please, call me John." Call him Jack, Jackie, or Jack-meister without his okay, though, and you've probably gotten a tad too intimate.

Give people their space. Keep a respectful distance from people when you're talking with them. The problem is that everyone has their own sense of how much personal space they need. The solution is to hold still. "Pick a spot and stand there," Dr. Elgin says. "Your companion will define how much space he or she needs by moving toward or away from you." Once they have mapped out their turf, however, don't violate it. In situations where there's a definite pecking order, take your lead from the person at the top. Also, if the boss is sitting at his or her desk, never move around the desk or sit on it—even if the boss has done the same at yours.

Protect your private parts. Among the many mannerisms singular to Americans is the habit of men resting the ankle of one foot across the knee of the opposite leg while sitting. "This nonverbal communication probably signals more informality than some people would like to express," says linguist Lawrence Davis, Ph.D., chairman of the English department at Wichita State University in Kansas. Especially in some foreign countries such as Japan, this would be a gesture of disrespect, pre-

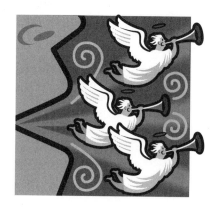

sumably because it showcases one's crotch area, says Dr. Davis.

Cover your dangling participle. Obey the rules of standard grammar "that are more or less accepted by educated people," advises Dr. Davis. "You'll stub your toe, so to speak, if you try to use anything non-standard." Also off-putting is when people try to mimic the style of the person to whom they're speaking. It would be a mistake to use "ain't" or "youse guys" with less-educated people, thinking it's showing them respect. "Trying to be something other than what you are is a big sign of disrespect," Dr. Davis says.

Play it straight. Part of body language is posture. "If you're hunched over, it looks like you're apologizing or you're hiding something," says Mary Mitchell, president of Uncommon Courtesies, a Philadelphia-based training and consulting firm, and author of *The Complete Idiot's Guide to Etiquette* as well as the "Ms. Demeanor" column syndicated to newspapers throughout the United States. So stand up straight. Also, don't fidget. People will assume that they are making you nervous—and you probably are if you're fidgeting.

Name names. Use a person's name when you're speaking to them. It will serve two purposes. In a first meeting, it will help you remember their name. Also, everyone loves to hear their name. Yessiree, Bob. And we mean you, Bob. Okay, Bob? However, don't overdo it (as we just did). "To get overly effusive is obsequious," Mitchell says.

Control the volume. Some people think that they command respect by speaking loudly. "Speaking loudly to make a point in a social setting is often counterproductive

---

Curses, Foiled Again

Using foul language can be a double-edged sword of respect.

"Profanity is often a signal that the level of discussion is informal," says linguist Dr. Lawrence Davis. "Or it can be used very much like certain kinds of slang to say you and I are members of the same group. 'How the f—— are you?' suggests we're connected." If that's the case, viewers of filmmaker Brian De Palma's 1984 *Scarface*, starring Michelle Pfeiffer and Al Pacino, must have felt very connected. That flick raised the use of the forbidden four-letter epithet to new heights—or depths. It was spoken 206 times, an average of once every 29 seconds.

Use profanities only when you already have a long-term, informal relationship with someone, Dr. Davis strongly advises. Casually dropping the F-word into conversation shows that the speaker is lowering his guard and regards the person to whom he is speaking as an equal, he says. "That could easily backfire on you in any number of ways if you don't know exactly with whom you're dealing," he warns. "Some people might consider them fighting words."

---

because you're drawing attention to the volume and not the message," Mitchell says. Other people think that speaking softly commands respect. "There's a big difference between lowering your voice and speaking softly," Mitchell notes. "Lowering your voice will get people to listen. Speaking softly will make them ask you to repeat what you said." How do you know when you're speaking too loudly or softly? If you notice them leaning too close to you, they can't hear you. If they step back when you pontificate, you're probably offending their eardrums.

Eating and Esteem

A Healthy Respect for Food

Friday night. Helluva work week. Now you're alone. No plans. Fine. Just fine—really. There's always the SportsChannel, a big bowl of spaghetti, and that six-pack chilling for just such a non-occasion. So you boil up a pound of pasta, top it with meatballs, marinara sauce, and mounds of Parmesan cheese, wash that all down with that brew, top *that* off with Cherry Garcia ice cream, and doze off to reruns from that first women's professional basketball season. Sad? Lonely? Depressed? Who, you? Not you.

Yeah, you.

"We can often tell when people are depressed and anxious by their eating habits," says clinical psychologist Howard Rankin, Ph.D., adjunct professor in the department of public health at the University of South Carolina in Columbia, founder and executive director of the Carolina Wellness Retreat in Hilton Head Island, South Carolina, and author of *Get Motivated, Get Smart, Get Slim.* "They eat more and worse. We tend to use food to comfort our emotions. And anytime you use something like food to protect yourself from your emotions, you're likely to do it compulsively."

In a study, Dr. Rankin found that men may indulge in bingelike eating habits when they're down on themselves as much as women do. But unlike women, who get upset with themselves for overeating, "men have been culturally educated to see big appetites as very manly." After all, we call rich men "fat cats." And remember your mom's declaration of pride when you ate everything on your plate?

Comfortably Numb

Food can definitely make you feel good. That may explain the popularity of what we've come to call comfort food. Sale of meat loaf, mashed potatoes, stews, and other styles of home cooking are on the rise, reports a survey sponsored by the *Thomas Food Industry Register* and the research firm of FIND/SVP. "The demand for this type of food seems to indicate a desire for dining options that make us feel good, especially in these increasingly stressful times."

But that comfort food can also cause us discomfort. "We associate it with being loved and accepted," Dr. Rankin says. "But it's usually rich, heavy, and high in cholesterol and sugar, so it sedates us and numbs us from feelings we may be denying."

But we know all this, right? So why then, after a long day of work, do even the connoisseurs of healthy cuisine among us reach for the frozen cheese steak instead of the low-fat TV dinner? "Because we want to reward ourselves for staying disciplined in other areas of our life," explains Dr. Rankin. "And we have been taught that rich, indulgent food is one of those rewards."

Regrettably, we pay a price for those indulgences. But the object of this chapter is not to wag a guilt-tripping, gravy-dripping finger at you. You know the dietary shoulda's. Eat your fruits and vegetables. Cut down on foods high in saturated fats. Fill up on fiber. Cool it with the excessive alcoholic indulgences. We're here to remind you to have a healthy respect for the effect food has on your body and mind.

Respecting food doesn't mean you have to entirely change your eating habits or your lifestyle, says Arnold Andersen, M.D., professor of psychiatry at the University of Iowa Hospitals and Clinics in Iowa City and editor of *Males with Eating Disorders.* "Along with moderate regular exercise, I

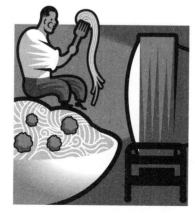

recommend eating in a healthy manner until you're no longer hungry, avoiding saturated fats (like full-fat dairy products and red meat) in excess, and letting your beautifully developed brain, rather than stress, control what, when, and how you eat," he says.

Eat and Run

Eating on the run or under stress is probably one of the most common ways we show disrespect for our bodies and total disregard for the debilitating effect food can have on our systems. Stress causes blood to rush to our outer extremities—arm and leg muscles—in preparation for anything from wrestling down a saber-toothed tiger to racing to catch a bus. That takes blood away from the stomach, where it's needed to help digest food. Gobble that burger and you're in for a whopper of a bellyache. *Hint:* Just because it's called fast food doesn't mean you have to eat it fast, advises nutritionist Evelyn Tribole, R.D., author of *Eating on the Run.* Slow down and smell the sandwich, and in the process, give your digestive system time to catch up to your lifestyle in the fast lane.

Many of us interpret that to mean we should skip meals rather than wolf down some grub. Here's the drawback to that side-stepping strategy: Meal-skippers don't perform as well. They accomplish less work, are physically less steady, and are slower at making decisions, Tribole says. People who skip meals have lower metabolism rates, which makes it more difficult to lose weight. Also, glucose stores in the liver are depleted within 3 to 6 hours if you haven't eaten. Consequently, the body will then begin to break down lean body tissue such as muscle.

Disorderly Conduct

Eating disorders, such as anorexia and bulimia, are most frequently associated with women. Part of the reason for the association is that eating disorders in men often are neglected by bias or lack of knowledge of professionals as well as hesitation or shame in boys or men, says Dr. Arnold Andersen of the University of Iowa Hospitals and Clinics.

"If a woman disappears to the bathroom regularly after meals, I think people wonder if she has bulimia," he says. "However, if a man chows down a six-pack and two pizzas and then throws up, it's sort of tolerated and passed off as guy behavior."

But, Dr. Andersen estimates, one in 10 people with eating disorders who come into his clinic are men. He cites a Toronto study that puts that figure at one in six or even higher.

"Many of the men with these disorders are dealing with a search for self-esteem, for personal identity, for meaning, and for relief from personal struggles that go right to the core of developmental and interpersonal issues," Dr. Andersen adds.

Bingeing and purging or nearly starving yourself to death are not the problem; they are just symptoms. Dr. Andersen recommends speaking to a physician or professional counselor to explore the deeper questions of how to get respect from others and how to give it to yourself.

"We don't want to make illnesses out of eating behaviors that are based on short-term stresses," Dr. Andersen says. But he warns that if there are consistent, long-term abnormal patterns of eating too much or too little, it's worth thinking about whether this is an unhealthy response to other stress mechanisms.

Fit to Take On the World

Respect Is for Every Body

If you're not motivated to stay in good physical shape for yourself, do it for the people you most want to respect you.

"I've found that the best predictor of success in changing behavior is when people are emotionally moved by people close to them," says James Loehr, Ed.D., president and chief executive officer of LGE Sport Science in Orlando, Florida, and author of *Stress for Success.*

That emotional motivation can ignite a radical desire to earn the respect of those you love by improving your physical appearance, which, in turn, will make you respect yourself more.

"Across the spectrum—whether you're a collegiate competitor or a recreational athlete—you're going to feel better about yourself if you're in better shape," says Steven Ungerleider, Ph.D., a research psychologist and director of Integrated Research Services in Eugene, Oregon; a member of the U.S. Olympic Committee Sports Psychology Registry; and author of *Mental Training for Peak Performance.*

In interviews with almost 600 competitive athletes 45 years old and up, Dr. Ungerleider found three key motivations: They love to compete; working out makes them feel better, and they enjoy being told they look good. "When we're in shape, people give us that external feedback," he notes. "But intrinsically we feel good about ourselves. We feel more energetic, more alert, more productive."

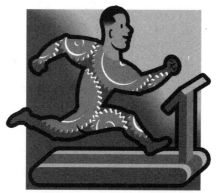

For those having trouble starting or sticking with a workout schedule, Dr. Ungerleider suggests dabbling "just to get a taste of how good you can feel." A quick way to remind yourself of the benefits is by doing some simple stretching exercises. You don't need to join a fancy-schmansy gym or buy expensive designer workout gear. You just need loose clothes and enough floor space to lay down and spread your limbs. You can even do it while you're doing something else—like watching television.

"Stretching is one of the great magic miracle workers," Dr. Ungerleider says. "It helps you stand up straighter; it gets a little blood flowing, puts a little bounce in your walk. It reminds you that you do indeed have a body and you need to respect it."

If you don't, it won't respect you back. As an added perk, stretching will help prevent injuries by giving your body more flexibility, Dr. Ungerleider adds.

For men, the relationship between fitness and self-respect is even more critical than it is for many women, says Steve Edwards, Ph.D., professor of sports psychology at Oklahoma State University in Stillwater. "The physical self is really important to men because we are so highly identified with what we do," he says. "And our bodies are the machines we do it with." Also, he adds, "we put so much value on appearance because 80 percent of the information we process comes from our eyes. If we didn't have mirrors, it might be a different story."

A large percentage of us don't start with the greatest respect for our machines. One study, by Thomas F. Cash, Ph.D., professor of psychology at Old Dominion University in Norfolk, Virginia, and author of *The Body Image Workbook*, found that 72 percent of the men surveyed said they were unhappy with some aspect of their appearance, while 20 percent zeroed in specifically on facial flaws.

Setting Goals

Aside from what you can do physically, Dr. Edwards suggests things you can do mentally in preparation for getting in shape.

Make your body matter. Elevate physical fitness to "a place of importance in your life," he says. "You can't just look into this metaphorical mirror, continually be upset with what you see, and not do anything about it." The first step, like anyone else trying to combat a self-destructive behavior, is to admit there's a problem. Then make rectifying that problem a top priority.

Arm yourself with information. Find, read, ask, research, discover everything you can about how to go about building the body you'd like to own. "Seek out information that allows you to do what needs to be done," says Dr. Edwards. That could be information on exercise techniques and equipment, aerobics classes, weight-training programs, weight-loss regimens, and other strategies.

Respect respectable role models. For women, the wrong role models would be those starved runway models. For men, it might be those steroid-infused mutants on the covers of many men's muscle magazines. "Be sure that the standards you're striving for are right for you, not the ones being sold to you by the media," Dr. Edwards says.

Following Through

If getting in shape makes an annual appearance on your list of New Year's resolutions, join the club. About 25 percent of those who make a resolution lose their resolve after the first week; another 25 percent drop out by the end of the first month, and by the end of June, only 20 percent of those who first made resolutions will still be committed to them.

Those bleak figures come from John Norcross, Ph.D., professor of psychology at the University of Scranton in Pennsylvania, who has conducted more than 30 studies of how people change their behavior. "Willpower does not come in a bottle," Dr. Norcross says. "Self-discipline is a series of behaviors that can be taught and learned." Here are several tips from him and others for staying with the fitness programs that will boost your respect for your own body.

Set achievable short-term goals. "Be realistic, not idealistic," says G. Alan Marlatt, Ph.D., professor of psychology and director of the Addictive Behaviors Research Center at the University of Washington in Seattle. Attempting to lose 30 pounds in 30 days is not only dangerous but it's also a set-up for failure and will only reinforce low self-respect, he says.

Replace bad habits with good ones. Those who succeed in quitting bad stuff do so by rewarding themselves with good stuff, Dr. Marlatt says.

"You need to be repulsed by what's behind you and attracted to the light of change in front of you," adds Dr. Norcross. "We have found that relying on either alone is not as effective."

Buddy up. There are two reasons that you should have a workout partner, says Dr. Edwards. One is the social pressure (a.k.a. the guilt factor). "It's harder to back out on a buddy," he says. The other is social support (a.k.a. the misery-loves-company factor). "When you see 20 other people working out alongside you, you feel you're in this together and you can get through it together," Dr. Edwards says. "Many wouldn't even be there if not for that built-in support system."

Recover from slips. Dr. Marlatt found that those who see a "relapse" as a "slip" from which they can recover have a better chance of keeping their resolve. Those too harsh on themselves quit in disappointment. "Be gentle on yourself," says Dr. Marlatt. "Avoid absolutes."

A Respectful Attitude toward Sex

Open Yourself to the Possibilities

What's a four-letter word for intercourse that ends in *k*?

Wrong.

It's T-A-L-K. Talk about yourself, talk about your real and true self. Not the I-did-this, I-own-that, I-know-such-and-such and what's-his-name monologue some men deliver. That's a sure turnoff, a bellwether of disrespect.

"The real turn-on that women desperately crave is an intensely private revelation of feelings from a man—a portal into his inner soul," says Robert C. Kolodny, M.D., medical director and chairman of the nonprofit Behavioral Medicine Institute in New Canaan, Connecticut, and co-author with William Masters and Virginia Johnson of *Heterosexuality*. "The starting point of respectful sex between consenting adults is the presentation of yourself in an honest and forthright way."

And then there's the kind of foreplay that involves the ears. Not the whisper-in-her-ear-and-she'll-follow-you-anywhere variety. But rather listening—*really listening*—to what a woman is saying. Not so that you can come up with some clever repartee in response, but in order to hear what her heart and soul are trying to tell you.

"The sexiest thing you can do is really pay attention when she's talking," says Bonnie Jacobson, Ph.D., director of the New York Institute for Psychological

Change and author of *If Only You Would Listen*.

If there were more of this sort of respectful sexual foreplay, there would be a lot more men and women walking around the streets with that telltale morning-after afterglow.

Honesty Is the Best Policy

The key to a respectful attitude toward making love to a woman begins way before intercourse. As with every other human relationship, it has to do with honoring the wishes and desires of your mate. "It's about treating others as you would like to be treated," explains Dr. Kolodny.

That starts with honesty. When you meet a woman, do you tell her you're not involved with someone when you really are? Do you say you want to be in her life when you really mean you just want to be in her bed? Do you say you've made love to only five women in your life when the truth is you're challenging Wilt Chamberlain's record (and we don't mean most points scored in a basketball game)? Do you whisper in her ear, "I love you" when you mean, "I lust you"? The next morning do you say, "I'll call you later" when you mean, "I'll call you when Elvis resurfaces"?

These are among the most common lies men tell women, according to Barry McCarthy, Ph.D., a psychologist at the Washington Psychological Center who teaches a course in human sexual behavior at American University in Washington, D.C., and is co-author of *Sexual Awareness.*

"Making promises you don't intend to keep is disrespectful," says Dr. McCarthy. "Don't oversell how much intimacy you want to have just to score."

Believe it or not, most women see right through that. Eventually, it catches up to you when she—and every girlfriend she talks to—catches on.

Along with honesty come

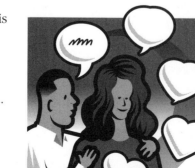

integrity, trustworthiness, reliability, and the other traits that distinguish the well-respected man. Then there's having the appropriate attitude. Too often men approach sex as something they "get." As in "getting laid," or "Did you get any last night?" This does not bode well for a healthy and respectful give-and-take sexual involvement. It implies that women are there for your pleasure.

"Sex is a shared experience," Dr. Jacobson says. "It turns out that the more you give of yourself, the more you'll get in return."

Regardless of your current marital status, there are basically three stages to the love-making ritual: before, during, and after. What follows are guidelines for each stage that will make sure you always show your mate the highest respect.

Prelude to Passion

So they want to see into our inner soul, do they? Well, some men take that idea to the extreme, dumping all their grief and vulnerability on an unsuspecting woman. If that's your version of sharing, go tell your shrink. "You don't want to dump," Dr. Jacobson says. "You want to connect." The way to connect is to "build a bridge," she notes. If there are serious subjects that you want to talk about—like losing a close friend—start by asking her if she has ever suffered any losses. Let her reveal some of hers. Then say, "Well, then you probably can relate to what I'm going through." Then share your grief with her.

If you've done this in a sensitive and sincere manner, believe it or not, you've just had great foreplay. Because great sex starts with great foreplay, and great foreplay starts with touching a woman—that is, touching her emotionally. Here are other ways to touch her.

Listen empathetically. There's no way to con a woman into thinking you are listening to her when you're actually listening to the hockey game on the radio in the background. "Women have a very sensitive

barometer, and they'll know you're only pretending to listen," says Rosalyn Meadow, Ph.D., a Phoenix-based sex therapist and author of *Good Girls Don't Eat Dessert.*

The giveaway is that you have a different look on your face; there's a different level of attentiveness in your eyes. Listening empathetically involves trying to understand what she's feeling behind what she's saying. "Enter her world," says Dr. Meadow. "Listen in an uncritical, nonjudgmental manner." Maintain eye contact. Resist the man's natural urge to jump in and solve her problems. If she wanted a problem-solver, she would have called her lawyer.

Plan unplanned time. This may be truer for married or committed men, but single men should take note, too. Allow unscheduled time and space in which "nothing has to happen," suggests Dr. Jacobson. "That's where real contact is made." That's when a woman knows you want to be with her for who she is, not for how good she looks on your arm at the opera or what you have in mind for after the fat lady sings.

Watch for love signals. Most men are oblivious to women's sexual overtures, says biologist Timothy Perper, Ph.D., a Philadelphia-based sex researcher and author of *Sex Signals.* In his research, he found that women initiate courtship gestures more than two-thirds of the time. At a social gathering, women will approach, talk, turn toward a man, and—most important—make physical contact in a subtle manner that goes right over men's heads. A light touch on the hand or elbow can be the female equivalent of a neon sign shouting, "Make love to me." It would show a woman great respect to let her do what comes naturally—initiate—rather than force yourself on her. And if she does not return your gestures—if she looks away, if she doesn't lean toward you—these are sure signs she's not into it, Dr. Perper says. The respectful thing to do is back off and let it go. Ironically, that sign of respect may win you points at another time.

Mean what you say. "It has to come naturally, from the heart," says Dr. Meadow. "If it's contrived or part of a strategy, it will come off falsely." And lying is no way to show respect. We suggest you read all this advice and file it in your subconscious, where it will take seed and later blossom organically as a many-petaled flower of love.

The Act of Love

You may think the sexual revolution began in the Summer of Love and ended in the Era of AIDS. But women are redefining their sexual needs in a worldwide gender revolution that's still going on in every one of 32 countries surveyed by Robert Francoeur, Ph.D., professor of biology and sexuality at Fairleigh Dickinson University in Madison, New Jersey, and author of *The International Encyclopedia of Sexuality*.

The new buzzword is "outercourse," he says, not intercourse. "Women are oriented toward the whole body, not just the genitals," he says. "They're redefining sex in terms of ecstasy. They want it to include a sense of transcendence." Talk about performance pressure. Now we have to worry about satisfying women spiritually as well as sexually. We have to make respectful love that makes her scream, "O-o-o-o-o..." and then chant, "O-o-o-o-o-m-m-m-m...."

This, too, is doable. Here's how.

Let her be the expert. Guess what? She knows what she likes better than you do. Rather than forge ahead caveman-style, let her take charge, suggests Dr. McCarthy. If she doesn't offer, ask. Or try something and ask, "Do you like this?"

Check out her breathing. Women start breathing faster and deeper and louder when they get aroused. Be attentive to these and other signs that she's having a good time. "Be attuned to the nuances of your partner's

The Not-So-Magnificent Seven

First, there were the Seven Habits of Highly Effective People. Now, we bring you the Seven Habits of Highly Annoying Lovers. Dr. Robert C. Kolodny, medical director and chairman of the nonprofit Behavioral Medicine Institute, highlights the seven sexual miscues virtually guaranteed to make your pillow your only bedtime companion.

1. **Play beat the clock.** On your mark, get set, wham-bam-thank-you-ma'am. Treat sex as a sprint, not a distance race. One sure way to let your lover know she's on the clock: Check your watch several times during foreplay. In fact, just wearing a watch is a good indicator.

2. **Take it oh, so seriously.** The "it's my job to make my partner happy" attitude guarantees neither one of you will have a good time. Furrow your brow, frown a lot, check the sex manual under the pillow to make sure you are following the instructions precisely.

3. **Be selfish.** Make sure you climax first, then "service" her after. If at all. This will go over really big. In fact, the whole relationship may be over if you use this technique too often.

4. **Welcome uninvited kids.** Children who pop into your room whenever they want to are the best

body," Dr. Kolodny says. The nonverbal cues, like heavy breathing, the slight sweat of her skin, and that musky perfume that exudes from between her legs—"vaginal pheromones," as Dr. Francoeur clinically calls the scent of a sexually aroused woman—are among the signs that you are demonstrating how much you respect her body.

Make variety the spice of your sex life. Send the missionary position on a retreat. Try it sideways, from the back, and other new variations on the age-old theme. Also, if the bed is your sole sexual arena, move the action to guarantee that you'll never have to worry about having more kids. It's just a shame there's absolutely nothing you can do about it. (Unless, of course, you count locks. Or hotels. Or sleep-overs. Or grandparents.)

5. **Make scents.** Just before you get into bed, smoke cigars, pipes, and cigarettes—all at the same time. That should be preceded by garlic-smothered pizza. (Don't brush your teeth.) Which all should be followed by a sweaty tennis match—hold the shower. The combined odor should leave no doubt you have no respect for her—or yourself.

6. **Bring your anger to bed.** In the 1989 film *The War of the Roses*, an estranged wife, played by Kathleen Turner, asks an attorney, portrayed by Danny DeVito: "Have you ever made angry love?" He replies, "Is there any other way?" Not that a divorce lawyer would relish. So if you want to turn a hot lady frigid, bring up past offenses as part of foreplay. Better yet, suppress your anger and let it out in sarcastic jabs.

7. **Bring stress to bed.** You missed the train. You lost the account. You spilled soy sauce on your silk tie. The annual budget is due tomorrow. You're losing your hair, gaining too much weight, aging before your very eyes. Bring all this worry to bed. Now try to get it up (we won't hold our breath). Then blame her for your impotence.

the living room or the kitchen or the garage. Wear your cowboy boots to bed. "The point is that even the most exciting endeavor can become boring," Dr. Perper says. Try something new; then in six months, when hanging from the chandelier becomes boring, go back to Position One.

Talk dirty—with respect. First, a warning. One style of talking dirty is using the most taboo of profane words, commands, and references to body parts that would make foul-mouthed comedian Andrew Dice Clay blush. The other is the more gentlemanly play-by-play

between consenting adults in which each thought and gesture is shared out loud—to the excitement of all involved. Some women love either style. Some, to put it mildly, don't. Dr. Perper suggests either letting her initiate the love talk or slowly introducing it yourself with mild obscenities like, "What a beautiful (fill in your favorite female body part here) you have." If she recoils, cease and desist, advises Dr. Perper.

Invent your own language of love. One of the problems with sex communication is that "proper words seem cold, and slang words seem hostile," says Dr. McCarthy. His alternative: Develop your own unique private sexual language. Make up vocabulary words that don't even make sense, Lewis Carroll-esque nouns referring to body parts or verbs for things you want to do to each other. "This is one way to personalize and individualize the lovemaking," says Dr. McCarthy, and to demonstrate to your lover the exclusivity of your relationship.

Avoid spectatoring. That's a term used by Georgia Witkin, Ph.D., director of the Stress Program at Mt. Sinai Hospital in Manhattan and author of *The Male Stress Syndrome*. It's a habit men have of checking out their own performance while they're still performing. It's like watching yourself through a camcorder placed on the ceiling. "Men have been performing all day at work," she says. "It's natural to keep doing it right into the bedroom." But it's damaging and impedes sexual spontaneity. Anyway, it pays more respect to your sex partner to let go of self-consciousness and focus on *her* body.

Get consensus. Now you're both involved in active sex play, but you want her to be in another position. Commanding her to turn over or move over may come off as too controlling to some women. Dr. Perper offers this variation: Gently push her body where you'd like it to be. If that doesn't work, say, "Do you mind if I move you over here?" This wording is key. "I've known a number of women who have explicitly described being turned on by that subtle demonstration of control and at the same time respect for and acceptance of her femininity," he says.

Put off the pouting. That sad look on your face, the Ringo eyes, and those curled lips when she says, "Not tonight" or "Not there" are "subtle forms of coercion" that have no sex appeal, Dr. McCarthy says. They may get you what you want that moment, but they will diminish your chances of getting what you want again. "You'll win the battle but lose the war," he notes, because she'll feel manipulated, and manipulation is disrespectful.

Have the condom conversation. In these times, unless you've been monogamous with the same person since the 1970s, contracting a sexually transmitted disease is not a remote possibility. It may be one of the most awkward moments in the dance of sex, but to show the highest respect to a first-time lover, you have to raise the question of protection. The most honest approach is the most forthright, says Dr. Perper. "Do you mind if I wear a condom?"

If you suggest it before she does, that is a signal that you respect her and you value both your lives. AIDS is a deadly disease, and this is no time to pretend otherwise. The where and when are up to you.

However, Dr. Perper suggests not leaving it to the moment before intercourse. That will deflate the moment and, quite possibly, your erection.

Truly Big Men on Campus

Almost one-quarter of college men admit to behavior that could be legally defined as rape, according to John Foubert, a sexual assault peer-education group advisor and Ph.D. candidate at the University of Maryland in College Park. And the single strongest predictor of whether a man will sexually assault a woman is if he believes that when a woman says no, she really means yes or maybe, he says.

"A lot of this behavior comes from socialization," Foubert says. "Men are taught from an early age to go out and get what they want, to be aggressive, assertive."

At Lafayette College in Easton, Pennsylvania, an innovative program started in 1997 is making great strides to reverse this early training of men, helping them to honor and respect what women want—and what they don't want. Called Coalition for Relationship and Rape Education (CORRE), it involves meetings of men and women as well as meetings of men only. Further, in a study involving 114 fraternity pledge class members at the University of Richmond in Virginia, Foubert found that 59 percent of the men who participated in a peer education program reported that they were less likely to sexually coerce women. They also were significantly less likely to believe "rape myths," such as that women falsely report rape to call attention to themselves.

After the Loving

For some men, staying connected after sex is not the problem; it's staying awake. If that's you, catch some Zzzs earlier in the day or get your beauty rest the night before. How you show love and respect after you make love is the sign of a truly concerned lover. So wake up and pay attention.

Make suggestions later, not sooner. The goal is mutually satisfying sex. If

Regardless of your educational status, you can earn extra credit toward a degree in respect for the opposite sex by following Foubert's lesson plan.

1. **Communicate openly during the sexual encounter. This has three parts. First, remember that cooperation doesn't mean consent. Just because she's going along doesn't mean she has agreed. Second, recognize what Foubert calls "the freeze." That's when a woman tenses up at your advance, a common sign that she doesn't want to go that far. Third, if she does freeze, stop, ask, and clarify. Ask, "Are you uncomfortable with this? Do you want me to stop?" Make a mutual decision as to whether you both want to get more sexually involved.**

2. **Get educated about rape. Do you even know the legal definition? Foubert recommends a book entitled *I Never Called It Rape* by Robin Warshaw. Or call a local rape crisis center and ask to be sent pamphlets and other materials.**

3. **Become part of the solution. Social change begins with you and your friends. Don't tolerate rape jokes. Interrupt other men telling jokes at women's expense. Sexist attitudes that demean women play into the rape culture. It's the man who doesn't fall into the trap of braggadocio and machismo who, "in the long run, will earn the greatest respect," Foubert says.**

she's not doing it in a manner that you enjoy, it's okay to tell her. When and how are the key issues. "It's better to not talk about it right after or during the interaction," advises Dr. Kolodny. "It sounds like you're a music critic and you're writing a review of the performance. That's one of the fastest ways to get a woman riled up."

Bring up technique at a time and place that's detached from that moment. Preface your suggestion this way: "I'm very nervous about bringing this up because it could sound like criticism, but I care about you so much that I want our sexual relationship to be the best it can be."

Clean up later. This is clearly not the sole domain of men, but some men who are a little too obsessive about cleanliness will jump out of bed and run to the bathroom to sponge themselves off right after orgasm. "It definitely takes the glow off the moment," says *San Francisco Examiner* columnist Louanne Cole Weston, Ph.D., a therapist with offices in Sacramento and San Francisco. "It makes a woman think her bodily fluids revolt you." If they do, discreetly bring a little hand towel to bedside and wipe off.

Cuddle. We all know women love to cuddle after great (or even not-so-great) sex. Why? It may be because they are more used to being cuddled as little girls, suggests Dr. Weston. It doesn't necessarily mean that they want to smother you or that they need attention all the time. If you jump up and grab the remote control right after sex, you're sending the message that your lover was interesting only as long as she was giving you pleasure.

"Women want a sense of continuity," Dr. Weston says. If cuddling feels too claustrophobic, or it makes you sweat, hold her hand. The main thing is for you to stay connected in a tactile way.

Brush your teeth. If you're a normal human being, your breath may not be worthy of being bottled and sold as perfume. If you're planning to kiss your lover in the morning or engage in face-to-face pillow talk, it would show great respect to sneak out of bed, tiptoe to the bathroom, and brush those pearly whites. "Almost every woman in the world would consider that a sign of respect," says Dr. Weston. And it might encourage her to do the same.

Respecting Your Elders

Tapping Into the Wisdom of the Aged

In other cultures, in other times, they are revered as the wise men and women of the community, the keepers of the flame, tellers of stories, the living symbols of continuity. But more than just human memory vaults, they are consulted on matters of great import. They are valued, even cherished, as sources of morality and inspiration. Others sit at their feet to understand how it was so that they can help pave the way for how it will be.

But that's in other cultures, in other times.

Rabbi Harold Kushner, author of the bestselling *When Bad Things Happen to Good People* and *How Good Do We Have to Be?*, says he finds it "hard to forgive America for setting the peak of life at age 25 and insisting everything is downhill from there."

"We're a youth-obsessed culture—we worship the youthful look," laments Debbie Then, Ph.D., a social psychologist based in Los Angeles who conducts seminars on health and fitness "at any age." Not only that, she says, but we live in a "culture that promotes getting older as something to be feared and dreaded." It's hard to respect someone when you don't want to have anything to do with them because they remind you of what you don't want to become: namely, old.

"There is no advantage to being young, except for being

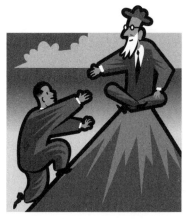

able to run fast and drink coffee at night," Rabbi Kushner observes. "Once you get over the physical first impressions, older people are more interesting than younger people. They're wiser, less competitive; they've experienced more."

For those who fear their best years are behind them, he suggests, "Rather than growing apprehensive about growing older, I propose we see life as the accumulation of treasures." He reminds us of this line from Job (12:12) in the Bible: "With the ancient is wisdom; and in length of days understanding."

"Every year with every book you read, every new person you meet and new idea you have, you have more life than you had a year ago," Rabbi Kushner says. "Then we can see the last part of our lives as the fulfillment of everything that came before it."

Now, Rabbi Kushner recommends, project all that on anyone you deal with who has a couple of years on you. It's the Golden Rule all over again: Treat an elderly person with the same dignity you would want when you attain that age.

Guidelines for the Golden Years

There's another good reason to respect your elders: There's power in numbers, and their numbers are growing. In 1981, people over 65 years of age represented 11 percent of the total population (25.6 million); by the year 2010, they will grow to 15 percent. By 2050, it could be as high as 25 percent. With such numbers also comes a growing responsibility on the part of the sons and daughters, grandchildren, and other younger relatives to provide respectful care when age takes its toll on the senior generation's body and mind. By 2020, as many as a third of American families will be caring for an elderly parent, predicts Thomas Humphrey, executive director of Children of Aging Parents, a national nonprofit charitable organization based in Levittown, Pennsylvania, which provides information and referrals for caregivers of the elderly.

For them and anyone else who has the privilege of hanging out with the aging generation, "The goal is to make them continue to feel useful and capable, and to maintain self-esteem and a sense of personal worth," says Michael T. Levy, M.D., director of psychiatry at Staten Island University Hospital in New York and author of *Parenting Mom and Dad: A Guide for the Grown-Up Children of Aging Parents.* Here are some guidelines for showing respect to your elders.

Involve them in decision making. A quick way to rob someone's self-respect is to take away their right to vote—especially when it comes to matters directly affecting them. Find the balance between taking care and taking control, Dr. Levy advises. The more you can involve an older person in deciding how they should live their lives—at home with their family, in a nursing home, with professional support—the more they feel valued and, incidentally, the more inclined they'll be to go along with the decision. It also takes you off the hook if they wind up unhappy about a decision they've been involved in making.

Be positive. Older people suffer losses almost daily: a friend passes, another memory disappears. It's too easy to dwell on those losses and get sad, so help them by concentrating on the humor and on what's good. "Make conversation light-hearted," suggests Lila Green, a lecturer at the University of Michigan Medical School in Ann Arbor and author of *Making Sense of Humor.* And never ask that loaded question, "How are you?" unless you really want to know and have time to listen. Instead, Green recommends asking, "What part of you feels best today?" Maybe it's only a pinkie or an ear lobe. "But this helps them by emphasizing wellness," she adds.

Go slow and low. Slow your conversational mad dash down a notch from 78 r.p.m. to maybe 45 r.p.m., suggests Green. Also, bring your tone down. "The higher-frequency tones are the first to go," she says, more so for women than men. She also recommends facing the person you're talking to; some can read lips, facial expressions, and other body language better than they can hear spoken words.

Unpack. Old emotional baggage—past pains and disappointments—can get in the way of both showing respect for your elders and taking care of them in their time of need. A son may find it hard to muster compassion for a parent who always favored the other son. Better to erase that stuff from your mind, Humphrey says. You'll have less anger and be less critical, more patient and forgiving in stressful times—of which there will be more than a few.

If problems do arise, Dr. Levy suggests calling meetings of the whole family to discuss plans. That helps avoid one-on-one confrontations; and accusations and blame can be spread around equally among all family members.

Exercise encouragement. Maybe their body hasn't been as good to them as they would like, but that's no reason for them to give up on it. In fact, that's all the more reason to encourage regular exercise, even if it's only a walk. "No matter what they have, it only gets worse with immobility," says Maryann C. Galietta, M.D., a member of the executive board of Children of Aging Parents and medical director at Statesman Health and Rehabilitation Center in Levittown, Pennsylvania.

Relive the past. Make a point of asking about important people and events in their lives. It would do them a great honor— and you might even learn a bit. You're also doing them a favor, suggests Rabbi Kushner, by helping them make order of their lives. "Life is like a good book that gets better as you get near the end," he says. "Only then do you begin to understand what it was about."

Winning through Losing

Having the Courage to Fail

Folk music fanatics will recoil at this, but we have to call 'em as we see 'em: Bob Dylan was wrong. In typically oblique lyrics from his song "Love Minus Zero/No Limits" off the 1965 album *Bringing It All Back Home*, he wrote, "She knows that there's no success like failure and that failure's no success at all." We take umbrage.

And so does Chicago Bulls professional basketball coach Phil Jackson, a guy who knows more than a little bit about success—and has the NBA championship rings as a player and coach to prove it. Jackson sat out the 1969–70 season with the New York Knicks because of a herniated disk. But that season on the bench served as the informal beginning of his training as a coach (which turned out to be not such a bad fall-back career).

"Losing is the ends through which you can see yourself more clearly and experience in the blood and bones the transient nature of life," says Jackson, a longtime Buddhist meditator. "Buddhism teaches us that by accepting death, you discover life. Obsessing about winning adds an unnecessary layer of pressure that constricts body and spirit and ultimately robs you of the freedom to do your best."

Taking a Risk

A man who loses his job, his marriage, or even his hair "enters a period of shock," says Dr. Warren Farrell, author of *Why Men Are the Way They Are* and *The Myth of Male Power*. "That period offers a window of oppor-

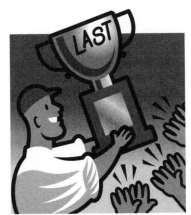

tunity to examine what his life's goals are." You can do that or get drunk, watch soap operas all day, and find a woman half your age who will deify you until she becomes too independent and dumps you back at square one again.

"They key question is, what do you really want out of life?" Dr. Farrell says. "Answer that, and the ways to get it fall almost naturally into place. I suspect if someone is reading this book, they have a good inkling of the answer."

Failure, defeat, disappointment, and other setbacks are the blocks that build character. It takes a winner to lose. That's not Zen mumbo jumbo. Losing means you took a risk. You accepted a challenge. Maybe you dove in over your head. But at least you had the self-confidence and the self-respect to try. You learned something about limits, about potential.

"The difference between being a winner and a loser in life is staying committed to yourself, staying tenacious, keeping the energy and passion high—despite repeatedly hearing the word *no*," says Wayne Allyn Root, chief executive officer of Root International, a motivational/business speaking and consultation firm based in Malibu, California, and author of *The Joy of Failure!* Root says he made hundreds of phone calls and failed at dozens of jobs before landing a newscaster job with Financial News Network Sports. He parlayed that into a lucrative gig as a motivational speaker and author and a beachfront house in Malibu. He suggests two other Fs that will toughen your tenacity: faith and family. "When things go bad after you've taken a risk, you want to have someone to turn to," he says, someone to give you another shot of confidence to get back in there rather than throw in the towel. Because the most important lesson of all, Root believes, is that "if you're not willing to face failure and rejection again and again, you will never succeed."

A Matter of Perspective

"We have to relook at the whole concept of failure," says Nancy K. Schlossberg, Ed.D., professor emerita at the University of Maryland in College Park and co-author of *Going to Plan B: How You Can Cope, Regroup, and Start Your Life on a New Path*. "Instead of being shamed by it, we need to embrace it. It's often through what we define as a setback that we are forced to re-examine and regroup." Here are several regrouping tactics she encourages.

Be thankful for what you have. There are many things we don't get. "If we start defining our success or failure by what we don't get, we're in deep trouble," Dr. Schlossberg says. She recalls a cartoon in which Snoopy, the Charles Schulz character, beats himself up for not getting an Employee of the Month Award. "Is Snoopy a failure?" she asks. "Not really, but he dwells on it so long that he sees it as failure." He could just as easily have thanked God (or Charles Schulz, in his case) that he wasn't fired from the cartoon strip altogether.

Conduct a cost-benefit analysis. What did you really lose in missing a chance to buy stock in pet rocks? How bad did tripping up the steps look on your way to accepting the Academy Award? Was she really the only girl in the world for you—poison fangs and all? Weigh the upside against the downside. In more cases than not, Dr. Schlossberg suggests, the loss will not be great, especially compared to the marginal win had you gotten what you thought you wanted.

Keep hope alive. In a study Dr. Schlossberg and her colleagues conducted, adult reaction to setbacks depended on whether the situation was hopeful or hopeless,

Born to Win

Vince Lombardi, the legendary coach of the Green Bay Packers professional football team, is often invoked when people start talking about winning. "Winning isn't everything," he said. "It's the only thing."

This desire to compete and to always win costs men dearly. In some cases, they pay with their lives. And we're not just talking about soldiers and sports heroes who die on their respective fields of battle. In a study at Duke University Medical Center in Durham, North Carolina, men who monopolized conversations, interrupted, and competed for attention were 60 percent more likely to die of all causes during a 22-year period than men who had a more relaxed style of communicating.

Nonetheless, we may well be hardwired to want to win. "In all the animal world, you will find that the entire male kingdom is characterized by extreme competitiveness," says clinical psychologist Dr. Howard Rankin of the University of South Carolina.

"Manhood is a test in most societies," adds David Gilmore, Ph.D., professor of anthropology at Hunter College in New York City and the State University of New York at Stony Brook and author of *Manhood in the Making: Cultural Concepts of Masculinity*. And what is the carrot that motivates men to want to pass that test?

"If you delve deeply, you'll find the reason is that they want material rewards," Dr. Gilmore says. "Why? Because that gives them prestige. And why do men want prestige? Because prestige, in their eyes, earns them the respect of other men and of women."

whether it occurred suddenly or gradually, and whether it was in or out of their control. Cut your losses—that is, don't dwell on defeat—when hope is dim, when it's out of your control, or when adversity happens so suddenly that there is no time to prepare. But make a new plan if hope still flickers, if you have the slightest bit of control over the outcome, or if there is time to fix what's broken.

From the Jaws of Defeat

You know the clichés. Turn lemons into lemonade. The difference between champ and chump is you. There are no problems, just opportunities. Here are five real-life ways to turn a setback into a success story.

Losing a job. Try not to take job loss too personally, suggests Richard Bolles, author of *What Color Is Your Parachute?*, a book that has enjoyed more than two dozen printings. "It's the nature of today's job market," he says. If you are fired, you will be in good—or at least crowded—company; in the United States almost three million people are laid off annually. The best way to deal with turning the loss into a win is to assume from the start that it won't last forever.

"Think of every job you get as temporary," he advises, and glean whatever information and experience you can from the time spent at that job. Basically, see it as a seminar and an adventure. Then, don't look back on it as a failure but as a paid chance to polish your skills.

Losing a love. She dumped you. You're bummed. The overriding feeling you're left with is that you will never find another woman to love you again. Ever. So rather than getting out there and dating, you spend hours at a time reviewing every conversation you and she had, every experience you shared, beating yourself up for the countless ways you failed to live up to her expectations. "Splitting up can stir humiliating feelings of having failed as a man," says Samuel Osherson, Ph.D., a psychologist at the Fielding Institute in Cambridge, Massa-

The Comeback Kids

Just think how much emptier our sporting lives would be if these immortals had quit at the first taste of defeat. And as you peruse their thumbnail bios, think about what *you* may be missing in life.

• Michael Jordan. The greatest basketball player in the history of the game unbelievably did not make the varsity team as a sophomore at Laney High School in Wilmington, North Carolina. In his video *Michael Jordan's Playground*, Jordan recalls that over the next year he worked very hard on his game, and he also grew 4½ inches, which didn't hurt. But he believes the relentless hard work on his game really boosted his confidence and determination. That determination led to NCAA and NBA championships and to the undisputed title of world's most famous athlete.

• Johnny Unitas. Coming out of St. Justin's High School in Pittsburgh, the future NFL Hall of Fame quarterback was rejected by Notre Dame and Indiana. After flunking an entrance exam at the University of Pittsburgh,

chusetts, and author of *Wrestling with Love*. He suggests seeing a split-up as an opportunity to establish or re-establish relationships with men and women friends and family, people who love you and will remind you of your positive qualities. You may have lost an important intimate relationship, but you now have a chance to win back and rekindle many other long-term relationships that feed your self-esteem just as well. In time, with patience, new love will appear.

Losing stuff. If you could total up the amount of time you've spent in your life looking for lost or misplaced objects and trade all of it in for a vacation, we're guessing you'd be gone for so long that your family and friends might start looking for you on the backs of milk cartons. "The lost time and money would embarrass most men," says Paulette Ensign, San Diego–based president of Organizing Solutions and author of the booklet "110 Ideas for Organizing Your Business Life."

Lose something really important one too

he went to the University of Louisville. Drafted in the ninth round in 1955 by the NFL's Pittsburgh Steelers, he was cut before he could throw one pre-season pass. On the tip of a fan, Baltimore Colts coach Weeb Ewbank signed Unitas, who at the time was playing for $6 a game as a semi-pro, for $7,000 on a do-or-die contract. His first pass as a pro was intercepted for a touchdown. But Unitas gradually emerged as one of the game's greatest clutch quarterbacks.

• **Connie Hawkins.** After leading his Brooklyn high school team to two New York City championships, this future NBA Hall of Famer won a scholarship to the University of Iowa in 1960. But he lost the scholarship and the right to play with any other NCAA team or the NBA when he was implicated in a game-fixing scandal, although no criminal charges were ever brought against him. After stints in the start-up American Basketball League, the fun-loving Harlem Globetrotters, and the upstart American Basketball Association, he reached a $1 million out-of-court settlement against the NBA. As a 27-year-old "rookie" in the NBA, he was an all-star with the Phoenix Suns.

many times, and the winning solution will hit you like a bolt of lightning. One solution is to tie things to your body, like Mom did with your mittens. Attach a watch fob to your wallet, or a short neck chain to your glasses. Attach keys to something so big you can't miss them. If you're the type who drops things in a trail as you enter the house, designate one place—a shelf or table or basket—right as you walk in the front door where you can unload keys, wallet, glasses, and toads from your pockets. Losing credit cards is a special case—a hellish nightmare, to be blunt. Create a list of all cards, with account numbers and phone contacts, and put it somewhere safe. Somewhere you won't lose it!

Losing self-control. Losing emotional control for many men often translates to fits and outbursts of anger. Contrary to popular belief and the frequent images of angry men in action-hero films, it does not win anybody's respect. And, in fact, it probably loses you several days of life. Anger kills, as many studies of anger-prone

men with high blood pressure and heart conditions have shown. The venting of rage pumps up the body's adrenaline, making the heart work harder—a true waste of beats. One way to win when people or situations trigger your anger is to turn that energy into constructive projects. But the first step is to recognize that something is making you mad, says Mark Epstein, M.D., a psychiatrist in Manhattan and author of *Thoughts without a Thinker.* "Note the emotion and its effect on your body," he says. That alone will help you begin to put some distance between you and the self-defeating emotion. Then take that emotion and invest it in something that will bring you positive results, whether it's a hobby, your work, or some physical exercise.

Losing the game. Being a sore loser at sports not only looks bad—John McEnroe throwing a temper tantrum on the tennis court was never a pretty picture—but it also hurts your chance of winning, says Dr. Steven Ungerleider, a research psychologist and director of Integrated Research Services. "Tennis is a perfect example," he says. "Investing energy in obsessing about the last blown point or game just makes you tense and tight physically and unable to focus mentally on the next point or game."

Dr. Ungerleider recounts the lesson Pete Sampras, a tennis champ who almost always maintains his composure on the court, shared with him. "Sampras told me that he'd continue to hold the image and the actual physical sensation of his stroke on a dropped point, which only reinforced in his mind and body the wrong programming," Dr. Ungerleider recalls. "Then he learned to just say goodbye to the missed shot, let it go emotionally, concentrate on relaxing his muscles, let his heart rate go down—basically to forget the bad, build on the good, and move on."

Earning Respect

The Fight to Regain Civility

The Comeback Kid commands everyone's respect. To beat the odds, to fall and then to rise again—that takes real moxie. To have had respect, lost it, and regained it— that is sweet victory. To make someone take a second look at you, your life, your accomplishments, and what you stand for— that very literally defines respect. The Latin root of the word combines *re* (meaning "again") and *spect* (meaning "to look")—or *respicere* for "to look back, regard." In other words, to look at again.

Basking in the glory of the comeback is part of every man's dream. On the football field, the legends of some of the greatest quarterbacks of all time—Bart Starr, Johnny Unitas, Roger Staubach, Joe Montana, John Elway, Dan Marino—are woven with dramatic come-from-behind miracle victories. On the battlefield, the battalion that courageously fights its way out of a death trap wins medals of honor. On the playing field of life, the man who takes on the task that others say can't be done—and does it—wins the corner office with the window.

Some men earn back our respect in such an extraordinary fashion that we must look up and take note. Tony Bennett, the 1950s crooner who was embraced by the MTV generation. Jimmy Connors, the tennis great who at 37 slammed his way back into our hearts. John Travolta, the dimpled cutie who disappeared after the 1977 film *Saturday Night Fever*, then reappeared in the dark 1994 hit flick *Pulp Fiction*.

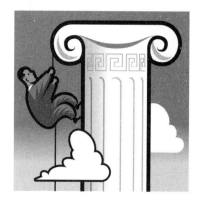

Respect Lost

Somewhere along the way, we lost respect. We lost it from others. We lost it for others. We lost it for ourselves. We've lost respect—as measured by trust—for those in power. A Roper Center survey in 1997 found that only 3 percent of the 1,500 Americans polled said they believed all of what is said by the President, members of Congress, and lawyers. We've even lost trust for those who report on the events of the day. The same study found that only 2 percent said they believe everything they're told by newspaper reporters, and just 5 percent totally trusted network TV news anchors (local TV anchors got a 7 percent trust rating, and radio talk show hosts scored a measly 1 percent).

"Americans seem to have forgotten the basics of civility," reports a 1996 "quality quotient" survey by Bozell Worldwide/*U.S. News and World Report*—civility being the first trait to get stripped away when respect fades and peels like a bad paint job. The report continues: "Its effects on society are serious, insidious, and far-reaching, according to an overwhelming majority of the public. Nine out of 10 Americans think that incivility increases opportunities for violence, while eight out of 10 say that it divides our communities and erodes moral values."

In terms of specific behaviors, according to the Bozell survey, 67 percent believe people are speaking to each other less civilly than they were 10 years ago; 72 percent say we drive our cars with less civility than a decade ago, and 76 percent say we are less able to keep our kids under control than in 1986.

In a 1997 survey by public opinion expert Daniel Yankelovich's DYG trend analysts, 87 percent of men and women reported a belief that morals and values have taken a nosedive. Ninety percent say family values have declined. And so goes the slippery slide of civility: Respect for others has declined 82 percent; honesty, 78 percent; loyalty, 75 percent; integrity, 74 percent; kindness, 69 percent; and patriotism, 62 percent.

Who's to blame for this unraveling of respect? "Not me," shouts a chorus of citizens. Only 1 percent report that they themselves are not civil, according to the Bozell study. Of course, the obvious inconsistency between that finding and the other reports on respect suggests that some of the people in that survey were not being entirely honest with their self-appraisal—or they were just in total denial of the ways in which they show disrespect.

Respect Found

So here are our choices: We can let respect fade into history as a nice idea whose time has passed. Or we can take the bull by the horns and turn this thing around. We advocate the latter. Reflecting the optimism in being able to control our destiny, in self-confidence and self-sufficiency—qualities in men the DYG ManScan survey tells us are out there in abundance—we can earn back respect, first individually and then collectively. And it begins with the next chapter, Self-Respect. In fact, all of part 2 of this book is a blueprint for the renovation of respect. Consider each of the next 11 chapters the pillars of the structure. Here's an advance peak at The House That Respect Built.

- *Self-Respect.* This is the cornerstone on which all other attri-

Jimmy Carter: A Model of Respect Restored

"Jimmy Carter has been a wonderful model for how to conduct yourself after leaving the highest office in the land. He's done remarkable things with his life," says Albert Eisele, the former press secretary to Vice-President Walter Mondale during the Carter administration who is now editor of a weekly newspaper, *The Hill*, which covers Congress.

Here's how.

- 1982: Jimmy and Rosalynn Carter found The Carter Center, a nonprofit, nonpartisan public policy institute in Atlanta dedicated to the promotion of peace and human rights.

- 1984: Carter volunteers for Habitat for Humanity, helping to build homes for the needy. He serves on its board of directors from 1984 to 1987.

- 1986: The Carter Center complex of four interconnected buildings, totaling nearly 100,000 square feet, is dedicated. It includes the Jimmy Carter Library and Museum.

- 1991: Carter launches the Atlanta Project, a community-wide effort to attack the social problems associated with poverty.

- 1991: The Carter Center becomes actively involved in assisting the international community to restore constitutional government to Haiti. In 1994, Carter joins a team that negotiates the departure of Haiti's military leaders. The Center continues to closely monitor the situation in Haiti.

- 1994: Following two days of talks with Carter, then-President Kim Il Sung of North Korea agrees to freeze his country's nuclear program in exchange for the resumption of dialogue with the United States.

- 1996: Carter leads a delegation to monitor and mediate the election of a new president in Nicaragua, which caps the efforts of The Carter Center in that country since 1990.

butes are built: honesty, confidence, integrity, and the rest. The bad news: If you didn't learn it in your childhood, it's hard to learn it in adulthood. The good news: You can work on it at any age in your life, and as you build on it, the other materials of respect will fall into place.

- *Altruism.* The Golden Rule is still the order of the day: Do unto others as you would have them do unto you. And, as you'll read, the good you do for others does you good, too. You don't have to quit your job and join the Peace Corps. There are many things you can do on a small scale to bring altruism into your life.

- *Cool, Calm, and Collected.* Men who are patient and have a relaxed attitude tend to live longer than in-your-face Type A's. The key to remaining cool under pressure lies in preparation, both mental and physical.

- *Confidence.* Here's the catch-22: To feel confident enough to succeed, you often need a taste of success. Here are two quick tips. Concentrate on your achievements, not your failures. And set reachable goals. Achieve them, then move on to some more challenging ones.

- *Daring.* We all have that little guy sitting on our shoulder saying, "I wonder what this would be like." Some of us just love that endorphin rush of the risk, whether financially, romantically, or from the end of a bungee cord. Others avoid it like the plague. If you're not naturally the daring type, you can still tackle dangerous assignments by crushing cynicism before it takes over your way of thinking. Look for inspiration in what you read, what you watch on TV or in films, and from the people you hang out with.

- *Honesty.* Here's how critical it is to the House of Respect: Lying can negate all of a man's good qualities. We still live by the code that a man is as good as his word. But that doesn't mean that we have to tell the truth all the time. This chapter will help you determine when a little white lie is okay.

- *Humility.* This trait is the one possessed by the "regular guy" who doesn't have to pretend, posture, or put on airs. How to do that without coming across as a doormat is what you'll learn here. Big clue: It starts with that first attribute, self-respect.

- *Humor.* A good sense of humor is the fourth most admired trait of the well-respected man, according to a survey of *Men's Health* magazine readers. It can also help you on the job front as well as with the opposite sex. Keeping a light attitude about life is good for your health, too. In addition, it's a great stress-reliever.

- *Integrity.* Perhaps the most difficult to define but the easiest to recognize. It comes down to the ideals of the Old West: a man living by a moral or ethical code that he will not compromise for anything. One expert breaks it down to three ingredients: deciding the right thing to do, acting on it, and then letting others know why you did it.

- *Trust.* Make a promise. Live up to it. Make a friend. Keep him. Make a commitment. Keep it. Make a deal. Honor it. Create expectations. Realize them. These are the pieces that slowly build a bridge from trust to loyalty, with a stop in hope along the way.

- *Wisdom.* There are smart guys, intelligent guys, wise guys—and then there are men of wisdom who combine common sense and some good ol' book learnin'. A little dab of both will do ya.

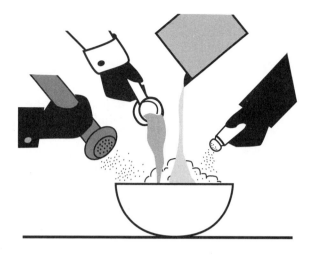

Part Two

The Ingredients
of Respect

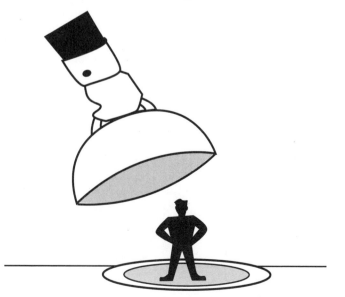

Self-Respect

Where It All Begins

Social scientists tell us that a first impression is made just 6 to 12 seconds after meeting someone for the first time. This, of course, follows a precise mental calculation that factors in such things as facial features, build, voice modulation, clothing, hygiene, political clout, and relative ability to impress chicks.

Underwear models, movie stars, and well-coifed TV anchor guys, naturally, score pretty high in this type of criteria. But it's the guys with self-respect—those who see themselves for who they truly are and value themselves from within—that generally make the best, longest-lasting impression. No matter how they fill out their overpriced, designer boxer shorts.

"Think about how striking it is to be around someone who genuinely feels okay about who they are," says Michael Nichols, Ph.D., professor of psychology at the College of William and Mary in Williamsburg, Virginia, and author of *No Place to Hide: Facing Shame So We Can Find Self-Respect.* "Most people shuffle along, head down...you can almost see insecurity written on their faces. It's the men who hold their heads high, make eye contact, and carry themselves with a sort of self-contained dignity that command our respect. By the way, that's why we admire certain movie stars—they project that kind of self-acceptance, that kind of self-respect."

Such an impressive, relaxed package stands in marked contrast to the many guys who feel like the quickest way to self-respect is driving a fire-engine-red Ferrari or living in a mansion in Brentwood. "It's

true: A lot of men spend their lives frantically looking for success on the job, huge financial rewards, the perfect spouse, these kinds of things, in an effort to build self-respect," says Mark R. McMinn, Ph.D., director of the doctoral program in clinical psychology at Wheaton College in Illinois and author of *The Jekyll-Hyde Syndrome: Controlling Inner Conflict through Authentic Living.*

Against the Wind

Although there aren't any studies that show how few men have healthy self-respect, it could be one of our country's biggest problems—and getting worse, says Nathaniel Branden, Ph.D., author of *Six Pillars of Self-Esteem* and *Honoring the Self: The Psychology of Confidence and Respect.* "I'll tell you why: Less is expected of people in terms of character or moral behavior," Dr. Branden says. "There has been a general falling of standards."

As a result, lots of guys have given into the Madison Avenue–inspired "He Who Dies with the Most Toys Wins" mentality. But creating your own personal empire, regardless of how vast and impressive it is, will never, ever give you the self-respect you crave. "Seeking or even achieving in this way is, in a sense, a Band-Aid to the deeper cries of the heart," Dr. McMinn says.

Nor does short-term self-confidence—the kind that you might use to pump yourself up for a sale or to get a job—improve self-respect. Sure, it may help you get over a career hump, or even win you a starting spot as a trash-talking NFL defensive back or American League outfielder.

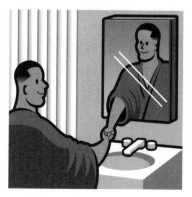

But arrogance or athletic ability should never be confused with self-respect. "If you're athletic, you're quite happy to step up to the plate at the company picnic. You have the skill, and you can rely on your abilities. But self-respect goes deeper than that. You don't have to perform," Dr. Nichols points out.

True self-respect not only gives us the freedom to "pursue satisfaction, the capacity for intimacy, and the ability to be alone," says Dr. Nichols, but it's also the cornerstone on which many other virtues—such as honesty, confidence, and integrity—are built.

That's the good news about self-respect: If you have it or are working on improving it, you're likely to develop other positive character traits as well. The bad news: If you didn't develop self-respect during childhood, there's a good chance that you're still suffering the effects today.

"Most experts think your home life is critical in the formation of self-respect," Dr. McMinn says. "Essentially, we learn to respect ourselves by whether we have experienced respect from others in the past."

Not to bash your parents or anything, but there are lots of ways they could have failed you in this. Chief among them: not letting you know that you were loved or accepted just the way you are.

Suppose, for example, that when you were a kid, you got the sense that you were only as good as your last finger painting or report card. No matter how hard you tried, you just never measured up. Such a performance-based environment can be murder on a child's self-respect—especially if those early renderings weren't exactly Picasso-like or gold stars were hard to come by. In fact, if this sounds familiar, there's a good chance that you've become a real achiever—but your success has still left you cold.

If your parents weren't as subtle, they might have just flat-out called you stupid, clumsy, bad, a mistake, or a disappointment. You don't have to be Dr. Joyce Brothers to figure out how much damage to self-respect that can do. Still other parents teach their kids to deny certain emotions—like, say, the sadness you should have felt when your grandmother

backed her Ford Fairlane over the family dog. And then there's the unmerciful teasing that some kids suffer at the hands of their peers—those hapless children who seemed to attract wedgies like a magnet. If any of those scenarios ring true, you may be settling for less than your potential because of unexplored feelings of self-doubt and inadequacy.

The Child Is Father to the Man

So what's the big deal—nobody's child-hood is perfect, right? We're not talking about perfection. We're talking about acceptance. "That's about 90 percent of it," says Dr. Nichols. "More so than spoiling us or even praising us. The important thing is our parents being okay with us as we are, not always criticizing and wanting us to achieve or perform."

Here's one theory about why that makes a big difference. When we're little people, adults are big, scary, and seemingly all-knowing—kind of like your boss down the hall. And we listen to what they say. If those big people continually tell you that you're bad, stupid, or whatever, you may have assumed that they must be right because, after all, they are big, scary, and all-knowing. The result is that it became a self-fulfilling prophecy. To prove them right, you flushed Barbie down the toilet, stole bikes, smoked, and generally ran amok, Dr. Branden says. And you may still be doing it today.

On the other hand, "children who do not feel their basic worth is continually on trial in their parents' eyes have a priceless advantage in the formation of healthy self-esteem," Dr. Branden says.

The bottom line is that whether you learned it from your parents or your peers, guys who lack self-respect are more likely to be intro-verted, hypersensitive, afraid of rejection, easily wounded, anxious, and timid. And they might try to mask their wounded self-image with arro-gance, rigidity, inappropriate dress, risky sex, drug and alcohol abuse, and overeating.

The Road to Self-Respect

The last thing that we want you to do with this information is to book yourself and your dear old mom and dad on one of those bizarre nationally syndicated talk shows and blast them in front of a crazed studio audience. And, of course, reliving your childhood isn't an option. But there are plenty of ways that you can build genuine self-respect into your life.

"The goal for all of us should be a self-respect so real that it saturates our human psyche, and in the process, we respect other people," Dr. McMinn says. Here's how it's done.

Make a stand. Whether you've cheated on your wife, stolen paper clips from the company supply closet, or any point in between, you can't expect to build self-respect if you're compromising your values. "There are some personal standards that we all have to live up to in order to maintain self-respect. And not just performance and achievement, but certain standards of loyalty or morality," Dr. Nichols says. Begin to live what you believe today—even if it's just that you think it's pretty smart to take a shower and wear a clean shirt once in a while. And if you don't know what you believe, it's time to start thinking about it.

Stop the blame game. It's so common that it's practically a cliché: We often hate in others what we hate in ourselves. "Anytime you hear someone nastily criticizing somebody for something, that is a concern of the person speaking," Dr. Nichols says. You can practice acceptance by learning to accept others as they are. And by the same token, accepting others is the first step toward accepting yourself, he says.

Pause to think. Next time someone says or does something that really ticks you off, take a deep breath and think about your response before engaging in what psychiatrists call emotional reactivity. In other words, flying off the handle. "This delay, this consideration, gives you the chance to respond more thoughtfully," Dr. Nichols says. After all, who commands more respect: a hothead or an even-tempered guy who thinks about what he says? "A definition of *assertiveness* I really like says that it's 'the straight-forward expression of thoughts and feelings that is socially appropriate and takes into account the welfare of others.' None of us could practice that enough," Dr. McMinn says.

Make "I" statements. The next time you're talking, count the number of times you couch your feelings in terms of "you" rather than "I." Instead of saying, "You don't give me enough feedback to do my job right," try this: "I need more feedback about how I'm doing so I can do a better job." Same basic message, but a whole different approach. Simply switching these two words does at least three self-respecting things: It helps put you in touch with how you really feel; it gives you the confidence to share those feelings; and it sounds more like your reasoned perspective than a lecture or criticism, Dr. Nichols says.

Take a long, hard look. Here's a suggestion that might be the toughest 15 minutes you've ever spent with yourself—and the most productive. Grab a mirror, a pen, and a piece of paper. Look in the mirror. Write down what you see—the good, the bad, and the ugly. "What's your best feature? How would you describe yourself to a stranger? What would be your first impression? How could you make a more positive impression? What is your worst physical attribute? How have you tried to cover it up? Now imagine a friend looking at that part of you. What would the friend say?" asks Dr. Nichols. As painful as it might be, the goal here is to help you learn to accept yourself for who you are.

Write for the silver screen. There have been a slew of big-time movie biographies over the past several years: everyone from Howard Stern to Nelson Mandela. But in the screenplay of your life, where does the story begin? Who are the heroes and villains? Does your main character—you—change and grow over the course of the film? After viewing your life story, would Siskel and Ebert be compelled to swear off movies forever? Or give you two thumbs up? "I encourage some of my patients to do this same type of exercise, with good result," Dr. Nichols says.

Make a list. For this exercise, compile a list of 10 words or phrases that best describe your strengths and weaknesses. "Then rank these characteristics from one (your most important) to 10 (your least important). How many of these are positive, negative, or neutral?" asks Dr. Nichols. Once again, you're getting a handle on who you really are.

Learn to jam. Some concert-goers prefer to hear their favorite songs performed exactly like they are on the album. But to break the monotony of playing the same song over and over, lots of musicians like to jam—also known as improvising. And that's just what you want to start doing with your life—especially if you've been timid and fearful. "Play is the freedom to go out on a limb with the knowledge that you might fall flat on your face," Dr. Nichols says. By the way, this could include—horror of horrors—finally learning how to dance, or at least cutting the rug once every millennium.

Jettison jealousy. Of all the possible vices known to man, none is responsible for more damaged lives than jealousy. The next time you feel the green-eyed monster growing in your gut, remember that it's rooted in insecurity about who you are. And that's an emotion that isn't compatible with self-respect, says Dr. Nichols.

Find a safe place to speak. After years of doing your best wallpaper imitation, you've decided to speak up for yourself. That's not a bad idea, but you may want to practice with really close friends or a spouse before breaking into your soliloquy at the next company board meeting. The risk of failure is high—especially if people aren't used to you weighing in on impor-

---

Instant Self-Respect

Let's face it: No matter how well-adjusted you are, sometimes you feel so low you could play handball with a horny toad. In times like these, it's a good idea to consider what some of the greatest documents in the world have to say about little old you.

The Bible: "Then God said, 'Let Us make man in Our image, according to Our likeness; and let them rule over the fish of the sea and over the birds of the sky and over the cattle and over all the earth, and over every creeping thing that creeps on the earth.' " Genesis 1:26

The Koran: "God obligeth no man to do more than he hath given him ability to perform." Chapter ii

The Declaration of Independence: "We hold these truths to be self-evident, that all men are created equal, that they are endowed by their Creator with certain unalienable Rights, that among these are Life, Liberty, and the pursuit of Happiness..."

Miranda warning: "You have the right to talk to an attorney...if you cannot afford to hire an attorney, one will be appointed to represent you..."

---

tant issues. "You need to be able to drop the facade and open up about certain things, like your weaknesses and insecurities," Dr. Nichols says. "What heals this wounded self-respect is exposing yourself as you are. And you need to do that in a safe place."

Make peace with your parents. There may be nothing harder, but trying to get closer to Mom and Dad will do two things: "It extends the network of sustaining relationships and overcomes unresolved emotional reactivity," Dr. Nichols says. "By going back to the source of our feelings about ourselves, we can make peace with the past and come to terms not only with our families but also ourselves."

Altruism

The More You Give, the More You Get

You've heard the expression "Give till it hurts." Well, it turns out that could not be further from the truth. Instead, we would posit, "Give till it feels good." That's the conclusion a host of researchers have come to. Consider:

• Volunteers appear to be physically and mentally healthier than nonvolunteers, and some studies have shown that they live longer, according to Mark Snyder, Ph.D., professor of psychology at the University of Minnesota in Minneapolis. And, he and his research colleagues found, those who get the most out of volunteering are the ones who stick with it. He identifies five benefits that volunteers attribute to their efforts: improved self-esteem, increased understanding of how others live, solidified community ties, affirmation of personal values, and personal development.

• Of 3,300 volunteers studied, 95 percent reported a physical "feel-good" reaction, called helper's high by Allan Luks, who was executive director of the Institute for the Advancement of Health when he oversaw the survey. Now executive director of Big Brothers Big Sisters of New York City, he co-authored *The Healing Power of Doing Good.* In his study, many also reported fewer colds, headaches, and backaches; improved eating and sleeping habits; and relief of pain from arthritis and lupus after doing helping acts.

• Volunteers 65 years old and older exhibited much higher levels of life satisfaction than nonvolunteers, according to a study by Norah Peters, Ph.D., chair of the department of sociology and anthropology at Beaver College in Glenside, Pennsylvania. This was true regardless of whether the volunteers were male or female or volunteered many hours or only a few.

• Even animals have a do-good streak, and it affects their brains. In several studies, Jaak Panksepp, Ph.D., distinguished research professor of psychobiology at Bowling Green State University in Ohio, found that a type of social interaction similar to volunteerism triggers the production of "feel-good" chemicals in lab animals.

If all this sounds self-serving—especially considering that we're talking about acts of altruism—it is. But that's okay. It's simply human nature, says Ray Bixler, Ph.D., psychology professor emeritus at the University of Louisville. Essentially, he says, "all animals are selfish." He calls acts of altruism sophisticated selfishness. Such gestures give a man "respect, benefits, status," he says. "It enhances your chances of being accepted and admired."

But this in no way tarnishes those who are generous with their time and money. Noting that "the most selfish volunteers end up making the most altruistic contributions," Dr. Snyder adds that "assuming that something is not altruistic if you're getting as well as giving is flawed thinking. It in no way diminishes what you are giving to other people."

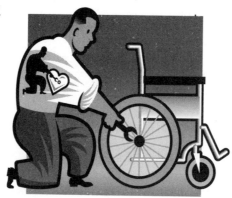

Making Your Connection

Put simply, altruism "is concern and caring for others," says Peter Dobkin Hall, Ph.D., research scientist and acting director of the Program on Nonprofit Organizations at Yale University's Institution for Social and Policy Studies. "It validates people's life achievements and careers. It gives meaning to people's lives. And it earns respect because other people reflect on the example of the genuinely charitable person and are led to act in the same way. And in that regard, it reminds us of the intricate interconnectedness of the community of Man."

Though church- and synagogue-related work is by far the most common sort of altruistic service, it comes in many shapes and forms: serving as a parent supervisor to your son's Boy Scout troop, contributing cans of food to a drive to help flood victims, helping out in a soup kitchen on Thanksgiving Day, responding to a multiple sclerosis telethon by calling in a cash contribution, donating second-hand clothes to the Salvation Army, attending a benefit concert whose proceeds support AIDS research, participating in a walkathon or bike-athon, joining an environmental group to clear a beach of debris.

Mentoring counts as altruism, too, whether it's done through such traditional organizations as Big Brothers Big Sisters of America, by taking on a young protégé at work, or by getting involved in a unique organization like CompuMentor, a San Francisco–based group that matches computer whizzes with nonprofit organizations that need help getting up and running with that funky used computer system someone donated to them.

"A lot of volunteers come to us feeling that there's a piece missing in how they're operating in the world," says Daniel Ben-Horin, founder and executive director of CompuMentor. "After getting involved, they say this altruism transaction completes the picture and makes them feel better about themselves and more whole."

Get Involved

If you want to get to work making the world a better place, there certainly is no shortage of organizations that need your help. Here are a few you can contact.

Big Brothers Big Sisters of America. With a total of 500 agencies in all 50 states, Big Brothers Big Sisters matches adult volunteers with school-age children primarily from single-parent homes. Can it help? A study showed that kids in the program were 46 percent less likely to start using drugs and 52 percent less likely to skip school. It also found that they were a third less likely to hit someone. For more information, contact your local branch of the agency, which is listed in the white pages of your phone book.

Literacy Volunteers of America (LVA). With 400 affiliates in 43 states and the District of Columbia, LVA helps combat illiteracy by providing one-on-one, student-centered instruction in basic literacy and English as a second language. Volunteers receive 18 to 21 hours of training in basic literacy or conversational English techniques and are then paired with an adult or teen student. For more information, look in your local telephone directory under "Literacy," or visit your local library.

Peace Corps. With a variety of educational, environmental, business, agricultural, and health projects in countries around the globe, the Peace Corps seeks volunteers from all professions.

Habitat for Humanity International. Through volunteer labor and tax-deductible donations of money and materials, this nonprofit housing ministry builds and rehabilitates houses with the help of the families that receive the homes.

Cool, Calm, and Collected

Prepare to Perform under Pressure

For the ultimate in grace under pressure, consider Bond—James Bond. No matter what the challenge—whether he's trying to rescue a bodacious babe or derail an evil genius's plan for world domination—007 always seems to emerge with the ultimate victory: hair in place and perspiration-free. (Reminder to self: Consider pitching "007 brand hair gel and after-bath splash" to merchandising.)

But when it comes down to it, a fair share of Bond's composure can be attributed to his trusty, white-haired equipment officer—the man they call "Q." It is this crotchety old chap, after all, who supplies the ingenious gizmos that consistently save Bond's urbane arse. In fact, you could argue that without Q's gadget pipeline—from radio-controlled helicopters and ejector seats to assorted laser-guided, exploding, bulletproof wristwatches—Mr. Shaken, Not Stirred would have gotten his clock cleaned sequels ago.

It would be hard to find a better example of preaching to the choir than telling a red-blooded American male that gadgets are the key to coming through in the clutch. But here's something that you may not be carrying in your toolbox o' tricks: mental preparation.

"The moral is that if you have your head right, that's when you can be cool and calm. You can know that you are going to go in there and nail it—whatever

you're doing," says Steven Ungerleider, Ph.D., a research psychologist and director of Integrated Research Services in Eugene, Oregon; a member of the U.S. Olympic Committee Sports Psychology Registry; and author of *Mental Training for Peak Performance.*

Going against Type

With apologies to Vince Lombardi, winning isn't the only thing—at least not when it comes to remaining cool, calm, and collected. A study of 750 men that looked at the link between personality and disease found that guys who exhibited what might be considered classic cool behavior—patience, a relaxed attitude, thoughtful speech—lived longer than the in-your-face, always-in-a-rush, highly competitive folks.

"The risk for Type A's is about the same as a moderate smoker and costs them anywhere from a couple to five or six years of their life," says Michael Babyak, Ph.D., assistant clinical professor of medical psychology at Duke University Medical Center in Durham, North Carolina. "At the root of it, Type A's seem to have a very basic insecurity about their ability and status and as a result are constantly, compulsively trying to be seen and in control. Internally, they are very fearful people."

While it once seemed that Type A's might one day rule the world, there's a trend toward cool-headedness afoot that may even land you a promotion. "People who seem highly emotional are viewed as less satisfactory employees," says Peter N. Stearns, Ph.D., author of *American Cool: Constructing a Twentieth-Century Emotional Style* and dean of the college of humanities and social sciences at Carnegie Mellon University in Pittsburgh. "Movements such as Total Quality Management urge managerial workers and

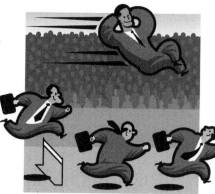

staff to identify and control vigorous emotions. They want people who are supportive of group harmony instead of those who would disrupt it."

Much of what we know about how to gradually change this kind of behavior originated in sports. But these techniques work anywhere for virtually any stressful situation. Here's how to avoid being a nervous wreck and, as a result, gain respect.

Select your skirmishes. Yes, life is a contact sport. But you don't have to smash everyone in your path, nor do you even have to compete with them. "Ask yourself: How important is it for me to win this conversation?" Dr. Babyak says. "Or better yet: Should I even walk around trying to win conversations and bowl people over? Such behavior is the opposite of staying cool—you're cranking out stress hormones all the time. And frankly, that's dangerous."

Feel the heat—and use it as fuel. You've finally found a worthy opponent, and the juices are beginning to flow. Your palms are sweaty, your heart is racing, and there's a sheepshank where your intestines used to be. Research shows that how you interpret this physiological arousal may actually determine your performance.

"If your body responds like this, you could either say to yourself, 'Man, I'm charged up and ready to go,' or 'Something is wrong,'" says Dan Gould, Ph.D., professor in the department of exercise and sport science specializing in sports psychology at the University of North Carolina at Greensboro. "You have the ability to view it as anxiety or a positive psyche, and it can make all the difference in the world in the outcome."

Enjoy oxygen. In other words, breathe! "Proper breathing not only relaxes you but also enhances performance by oxygenating your

---

Patience Place

When it comes to keeping your cool, patience truly is a virtue. Here are some practical ways to play the waiting game, courtesy of Kate Wachs, Ph.D., founder and director of The Relationship Center in Chicago.

Be a thought-stopper. The next time you're in the midst of giving someone a mental body slam for moving too slowly, instead practice what's called thought-stopping. Simply tell yourself to stop it, and move on to the next thought, like planning what you're going to do next or wrestling with one of those thorny problems you keep ignoring.

Ask for help. Lots of us have the mistaken belief that pounding our fists and demanding our rights will help us get better service and more respect. But assertiveness is one thing; acting like a loud-mouthed jerk is another. Even better: asking politely for help. Service personnel and other hired hands respond to this technique because they—and everyone else in the world—would rather feel like they're doing a favor than being forced against their will to do something.

Lend a hand. Instead of bellyaching, why not put your energy into lending a hand? That grocery store line will move a heck of a lot faster if you help the lady in front of you bag. And what can be more respectful than helping someone out?

---

blood and energizing your brain," says Dr. Ungerleider. Since breathing right is one of the first things we stop doing properly when we're stressed, it pays to practice deep breathing at least once a day. Start by filling your lower abdomen with air as if it were a balloon. Gradually allow the air to also fill your middle abdomen and chest. Then breathe out, says Dr. Ungerleider. See? That wasn't so hard. And you probably feel calmer already.

Make a fist. Not to pound people, tough guy, but to experiment with progressive relaxation. Now it may sound like something a swami would suggest between servings of alfalfa sprouts, but progressive relaxation is just another way of describing the process of tightening and relaxing your muscles. Start right now by making a fist and squeezing it for 10 seconds. Now relax and feel the tension drain away. Applied to the rest of your muscles—either before or in the heat of battle—that same concept can help put you at ease, Dr. Ungerleider says.

Be a doom-buster. Whether it's in the boardroom or on the basketball court, we're all bombarded by negative thoughts that can make us nervous and edgy. But you can put the brakes on these notions of doom by keeping a list handy of all the reasons that you should succeed. "One power lifter I was working with had a list of the 10 reasons he should do well at nationals, even if he didn't feel right," Dr. Gould says. Some of the items on the list included: I've trained well; I'm really strong even on my weakest days; and my technique is better than ever. "It may sound gimmicky, but the list is based on reality—not just a bunch of positive affirmations, which I'm not convinced are of a whole lot of value," Dr. Gould says.

Quit complaining. Maybe you remember a *Saturday Night Live* skit featuring a family of malcontents called The Whiners. In case you missed it, their shtick was complaining about everything—in voices so annoying that you truly understood for the first time what compelled Elvis to shoot out his TV. We all know people who adopt this kind of behavior at the first sign of trouble. If this describes you, wonder no more why you don't get any respect.

"Let's say your plane is late and you're

Acting Calm

Few experience the confidence-busting effects of rejection more often than an aspiring actor. Yet to keep the dream alive, actors not only must persevere but also thrive (unless, of course, they're content to do antacid commercials).

Such situations call for something remarkably close to what might be called instant calm. And to find out how the pros settle themselves before and during a big audition, we turned to Santa Monica, California, acting coach Larry Moss, who has coached such actors as Jason Alexander, Helen Hunt, and Paul Reiser.

Exude confidence. Whether you're trying out for a part in *Hamlet* or applying for a job in a hardware store, remember to feel like you're bringing something valuable and creative to the table. "It shouldn't be, 'I hope that you like me,'" says Moss. "It's two adults meeting on a project and deciding to work together."

Feel your feet. When people get scared, blood liter-

going to miss a meeting. You could sit there and complain and make everyone around you miserable, or you could take out your laptop and get some work done. And when the battery in your laptop dies, you could complain. Or you could borrow some paper and write out what you were working on. Or just catch up on some sleep. It's called making the best of the situation, and it's infinitely more healthy," Dr. Gould says.

Make adversity your ally. It's one thing to learn how to go with the flow—and frankly, that would be a big improvement for a lot of us. But another step toward being cool, calm, and collected is actually expecting the unexpected. "The really good athletes are prepared to cope with adversity," says Dr. Gould. "They realize that in sports people make ally begins to recede from their hands and feet. To nix this unsettling feeling, feel your feet on the floor and take a deep breath. "Acting is about being present in the moment, and you fail when you are outside the moment," Moss says. "But I think that's true with anything: business, sports, writing. You need to be present and stay there."

Change your focus. A huge part in the battle to maintain your calm is not thinking too much about yourself. That's why it's a good idea to focus on the names of the people you're meeting, watch their body language, or even check out the furnishings in the room. "You're trying to keep the energy on something other than yourself," Moss says.

Let go if you don't get it. Okay, so you're not going to be on *Seinfeld* this season. There's always next year—if you keep your attitude right. "The most important thing for an actor to know is that they're not what they do. That feeling that I failed and I'm not valuable if I don't get the job is completely antithetical to creativity," Moss says.

are called cue words written on the tips of their skis that remind them of what they are about to do. "They're very simple—things like 'Twist' and 'Turn and Go,'" says Dr. Gould. "They read that, and it helps them refocus on what they're about to do." You can place yours on your bathroom mirror, office bulletin board, or anywhere you need an instant reminder to stay calm.

Hang tough. We all have days—heck, maybe even a decade or two—that we wished we had just stayed in bed. Guess what: Guys who are cool to the core know this. And even when they are having a really bad day, they're banking that if they can just hang in there, you're going to falter and they're going to come out on top—again.

"Instead of really, really getting down on myself and kind of dropping into a Grand Canyon of failure where nothing goes right, I fight it and try to keep control—the best control I can under the circumstances," Dr. Gould says. "I have a bad day, but I don't have a disaster. And so when the bottom drops out on someone else, I end up winning ugly."

bad calls. Or they get injured. Or the weather just isn't right." So how does that apply to you? You may not be able to control whether you're going to get laid off, but you can make sure that you find the best job recruiter in the area. Or talk to people who have also lost their job recently and find out what they've learned. And then make sure that you work just as hard—or even harder—getting a job as you did at your old job.

Get a cue. It doesn't get much hairier than hurtling down the side of a mountain toward a giant ramp that will propel you hundreds of feet through the air—all with the expectation that you won't be imbedded in said mountain upon return. So how do some of the top skiers and aerialists avoid stressing out before their big jump? They have what

Go to a game. We all know that frequent exercise is a great way to blow off steam and keep the head clear. But raising cain at a Miami Hurricane game—or any other big-time spectator sport—is a great way to release pent-up emotions that can otherwise leave you nasty, brutish, and in short, the opposite of cool, calm, and collected.

"We let athletes do all sorts of things that we don't let ourselves do," Dr. Stearns says. "They can hug each other. They can dance triumph dances over a fallen opponent. It's not the best way to experience this kind of release, but for some of us, it's the closest we'll get." Do not, under any circumstances, however, wear a block of cheese on your head.

Confidence

How to Score the Winning Goal

In the never-ending quest to improve workers' productivity—the old more-widgets-per-hour routine—researchers have spent countless hours investigating goal setting. As it turns out, what works for the widget-makers can also work for building confidence.

"One thing I've argued is that people working in industry aren't particularly motivated," says Robert Weinberg, Ph.D., a sports psychologist who coaches several professional athletes and is chairman of the department of physical education, health, and sport studies at Miami University in Oxford, Ohio. "Yet goals provide them with motivation and focus, and when they achieve them, confidence. They know they can do it."

Knowing that you can do something—and do it well—is one of the keys to confidence. But there is a price to pay for that knowledge.

"Everyone wants to win, but you're not going to build your confidence until you experience some success. And any kind of consistent success isn't going to come until you pay your dues," says Dr. Dan Gould of the University of North Carolina.

Becoming a Confidence Man

A study of *Men's Health* magazine readers found that confidence ranked ahead of assertiveness, patience, communication skills, and ambition as the one characteristic that guys felt would earn more respect from others.

It also ranked second—behind only patience—on the

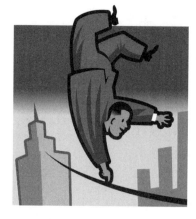

list of traits they felt they needed to work on most. And with good reason. "Confidence will allow whatever abilities you have to shine and really come forth," Dr. Weinberg says. "It's very, very powerful."

So why are some guys completely devoid of confidence and the rest of us wishing we had more? A large part of the problem is that Greek chorus of voices in your head reminding you of past failures and telling you that you're no good, Dr. Weinberg says.

"If you say, 'I can't do that. I'll never win this 10-K race. I'll never be a vice-president. I'll never get this report done'...whatever it is, you are telling yourself that you can't do it, and it becomes a self-fulfilling prophecy," Dr. Weinberg says.

To gain confidence, you have to set goals. Here's what the experts suggest.

Be a man with a mission. Before you even think about setting goals, you should spend some quiet time with yourself deciding what's truly important to you. "I can set a lot of specific goals that will help me get up the hill, but I want to make sure it's the right hill," Dr. Gould says. "It's like, 'Okay, what mountain do I want to climb?' "

Ink it, don't think it. Research shows that the simple act of writing down your goals exponentially increases your commitment level—a prime factor in helping you achieve them. "If I'm not committed to a goal, then what do I have? Statements that may or may not occur," says Dr. Weinberg. "Write your goals down, and watch your achievements go up. It works."

Make it specific and measurable. Someone once said that a goal is a dream with a deadline. And research shows that the best goals are exactly that. "Saying, 'I'd like to lose some weight over the next six months' is not a good goal," Dr. Weinberg says. "You want to have something you can measure. It's much better to say, 'I want to lose 25 pounds in the next six months.' Then you have something to shoot for and can see whether you are moving toward it."

Step on the scale. Rating your performance can help you meet more subjective goals, such as improving your concentration, says Dr. Gould. "I just rate myself on a scale from one to 10. How was my concentration today at practice? And that makes you aware of it."

Keep it short. Breaking bigger goals into smaller weekly and daily goals is another proven way to build confidence. "Making the Olympic team in four years sounds like an awesome challenge," Dr. Weinberg says. "But if I can do something today or this week to help make it happen, that's a short-term goal providing feedback as well as reinforcement on my way to the bigger goal."

Make goals challenging, but realistic. People who set unrealistic goals don't reach them, says Dr. Weinberg. "Your New Year's resolution might be that you're going to exercise five days a week. But soon you miss a day and you say to yourself, 'To heck with it. I guess I can't do it,' and then you drop it. But how realistic is it for anyone to exercise five days a week?" Goals set too low, on the other hand, fail to satisfy as well, he says. "You want to push yourself, but somewhere in the realm of your abilities," Dr. Weinberg says.

Keep an eye on the prize. Neat freaks and pack rats pay attention: Tossing your freshly minted goals in a desk drawer won't do. "Post them over your bed or in a place that you can see them every day—even several times a day—so you can remind yourself of what you're supposed to be doing," says Dr. Weinberg.

Spend Sunday setting new goals. Before the week is lost in a blur of events, take some time on Sunday reviewing last week's successes and planning this week's goals. "The question you want to ask yourself is, 'What do I need to do specifically this week?' " says Dr. Gould.

Other Confidence-Boosters

Both performance accomplishments and goal setting are great ways to turbo-charge your confidence. But there are others. Here's some more expert advice.

See your success. Basketball players talk about visualizing the winning shot leaving their hands and swishing through the net; sales guys see themselves overcoming objections and making the sale. Whatever form it takes, visualization can help make it happen. "There are data that show that mental imaging can enhance performance, and there are recent data that show that confidence can be an intermediary link, so that my imaging increases my confidence and confidence increases my performance," Dr. Weinberg says.

Hit the gym. One study showed that 77 percent of men feel more confident when they're in shape. Lift weights, run, bike, walk—whatever. But get some exercise that you enjoy at least three times a week for a half-hour or more.

Get a hero like you. When George Foreman won the heavyweight championship of the world at age 45, it served as a wake-up call to a lot of guys who had meekly accepted the conventional wisdom that they were past their prime. You may not be ready to step into the ring, but learning from others who have accomplished goals similar to your own can help you go the distance. "There's a confidence in looking at others, particularly others you respect who have some similarity to you," Dr. Weinberg says. "And seeing them doing something or performing can fuel some of your own confidence."

Get a coach. We're not talking about Rick Pitino or Jimmy Johnson here, but having a friend, parent, teacher, or colleague who's willing to encourage you can help you build self-confidence. "It's having someone in your corner saying, 'Hey, you can do it. I know you can. Just hang in there,' " says Dr. Weinberg. "Obviously, the more respect that person has in your eyes, the more weight they will have in building that sense that you can do it."

Daring

When Respect Gets Risky

Copernicus, Benjamin Franklin, Gloria Steinem, Bill Gates, and Madonna all share two things in common. (Relax: Neither has anything to do with undergarments.) First, they were risk-takers, daring to be different and willing to blaze new trails. And second, none of them was first—at least not when it came to birth order.

The degree to which you are willing to risk life and limb, like so many character traits, seems to be deeply rooted in childhood. But this time, it may have as much to do with *when* your folks had you as *how* they raised you.

"As best we can tell, first-born children are under-represented in risk-taking activities," says Arnold LeUnes, Ed.D., professor of sports psychology at Texas A&M University in College Station. "The theory is that they get their gratification, their pats on the back, from more conventional kinds of things like schoolwork because they are often the favored child."

"Later borns" often seem to have an overwhelming desire to prove themselves in less conventional ways. This desire also seems to translate into more "individualistic" behavior—which means they're self-motivated, entrepreneurial, and more comfortable with one-on-one competition than team sports, says Michael Meyers, Ph.D., associate professor of exercise physiology at the University of Houston.

And when it comes to respect, the guys who are willing to take chances, to break new ground, rank near the top. "I think down deep there is a spark in all of us that says, 'I wonder what this would be like,'" Dr. Meyers says.

The Endorphin Surge

Not that all risk taking is good. Sure, sometimes we're held back by doubt, fear, experience, or peer pressure. But sometimes, it's just plain old common sense. For example, Dr. Meyers says he has studied people who bungee jump, "but I have absolutely no desire to try it. There is one alternative for success and 10 alternatives for failure, and I don't like the odds. Why would someone want to jump off a perfectly good bridge?"

Why indeed. But it isn't just birth order or even common sense that determines your willingness to engage in daring behavior. Some experts feel it could be caused by a deficiency of brain chemicals. A shortage of endorphins, or so the theory goes, may drive a guy to cliff diving—or some other risky behavior—for a quick, natural high. "Any time that you get that beta endorphin surge, you're getting a feeling of euphoria. It's almost like you're taking a pharmaceutical drug," Dr. Meyers says.

And like most drugs, it's tough—once you've tried it—to just say no. "You can get addicted to the endorphin rush, so you'll have to do something to continue to get that surge—which could bring you to further or more extreme challenges," he says.

Add Some Daring to Your Day

Unless you're "Evel" Knievel, or his motorcycle jumping son, Captain Robbie Knieval, you're

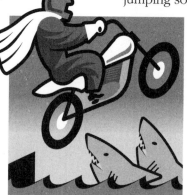

not going to need massive amounts of in-your-face daring-do to get through the day. But just in case you feel like life is passing you by, we talked to a self-made millionaire, a member of the New York Police Department's (NYPD) elite emergency squad, and one of the top stuntmen in Hollywood. Here are their suggestions to add some thrills, while minimizing risks.

Write your own obituary. If you were going to die tomorrow, would people say this: "That Ned really enjoyed eating bologna sandwiches and watching pro bowling on the tube." Or this: "You have to hand it to Chad. He never took no for an answer. Who would have thought he would try to climb the Himalayas again—at age 83?" If you could write your own obituary, how would it read? Wayne Allyn Root, chief executive officer of Root International in Malibu, California, and author of *The Joy of Failure!,* offers this advice: "Once you write your obituary, then work backward. Figure out how to live life in such a way that people could say that about you. If you want them to say you are a good boss and you're only an employee, let's figure out a game plan to get you your own business. That has to get you out of your chair and into the game of life."

Use the buddy system. Whether rappelling from a helicopter onto the roof of the World Trade Center after the 1995 bombing, or digging through the wreckage of the Federal Building in Oklahoma City, the NYPD's Emergency Services Unit has helped mount some of the most daring rescue operations in recent memory. Needless to say, rappelling onto the roof of a bomb-damaged building has a way of spiking the adrenals. But before anyone goes anywhere, the elite, 383-member squad uses a buddy system to make sure that all the ropes are sturdy and properly secured. In fact, similar equipment checks just prior to any rescue are the rule, not the exception, says Captain Curt Wargo, the unit's executive officer. In the same way, it pays to check in with a buddy or pal before making a big move— whether you're planning an extremely rugged mountain-bike trip or thinking about asking for a raise. A friend can help catch important things

Take the Plunge

During his successful run for the presidency back in 1988, George Bush—who was never known as Mr. Charisma—asked an interviewer, "What's wrong with being a boring kind of guy?" Yet here he was, at the age of 72, parachuting from a plane into the Arizona desert in 1997. Not exactly something a boring guy would do.

An aide to the former president told reporters that Bush hoped the jump would help give him closure from his World War II experiences. A fighter pilot, Bush was attacking a Japanese radio station when his Avenger torpedo bomber came under fire. Two crewmates died as Bush narrowly parachuted to safety.

Only Bush knows whether he successfully closed that chapter of his life. But don't be surprised if you see him take more risks in the future. There's evidence that cranking up your adrenaline once in a while can help launch even an out-of-work Republican (Motto: "Will cut taxes for food") into some challenging new directions— and as a result, garner some newfound respect.

that you may have overlooked—or are even trying to ignore.

Break it down. A second unit stunt director, stunt coordinator, and stunt double for Mel Gibson, Mic Rodgers has set himself on fire, rolled cars, and jumped out of buildings. But as Rodgers points out, stuntpeople who know their stuff understand that every blockbuster stunt is actually a series of much smaller maneuvers. "One stunt might be broken down into 10 or 15 littler stunts. The goal is to take most of the risk out of it," Rodgers says. If your life seems like it's imitating a disaster film (Hey, isn't that Shelley Winters over there?), there's no reason that you can't take your biggest problem and turn it into bite-size chunks of opportunity.

Honesty

To Tell the Truth

It is one of life's sweet ironies, a cosmic comeuppance if there ever was one: Respect gained through lies, deceit, and betrayal all but vanishes when the truth finally comes out. At least that's the impression you get when you consider the results of several studies that explored the qualities of a man who truly commands respect. For example, when posed with this question: "Are there any qualities so bad that they negate all of a man's good qualities?" the most frequent answer for 600 *Men's Health* magazine readers was "lying/dishonesty."

Of course, being against dishonesty is a little like being against acid rain, chemical weapons, or the Dallas Cowboys—you have plenty of company. Whether it's blatant lying by celebrities accused of crimes or convenient memory lapses by power-hungry politicians, the nation seems weary of such falsehoods and fabrications. Says Jim Lichtman, an ethics specialist based in Palm Desert, California, and author of *The Lone Ranger's Code of the West*: "There have been more ethics scandals in the last five years than in the last 50 years combined. And it's not just the big ones that you see in the news and get the big headlines, because everyone hears about those. It's everyday stuff...and it's appalling."

But while headlines may detail the dilemma and explain the outrage, they don't tell us why we lie—and how we can lead more honest lives.

Why Do We Lie?

Oddly enough, sometimes lying just seems like the right thing to do—especially when there's a chance that our friend-

ships or jobs are on the line. One study showed that 20 to 33 percent of employees in the past year have lied to or deceived a superior in order to make a supervisor look good or meet a production quota, or simply because it was easier, Lichtman says. Nearly 15 percent of top executives—those making $100,000 plus—lie on their résumés about their education, according to Jude Werra, owner and president of Werra and Associates, an executive search firm in Brookfield, Wisconsin. "And those are just the easiest ones to catch because you can check with a phone call," says Werra.

Altruistic lies—"the ones where you say, 'Oh, you look nice' or, 'What a great dinner'—show you're emotionally supportive," says Bella M. DePaulo, Ph.D., psychology professor at the University of Virginia in Charlottesville.

Falling somewhere in between the truth and a lie is exaggeration. It's kind of the truth, only, to use the advertising lingo, new and improved. Like when you regale your co-workers with the tale of how you barged right into the president's office, slammed your fist on his desk, and demanded—in no uncertain terms—that pay raise you'd earned. When, in fact, you nervously shuffled in and stammered your request in the politest terms possible, bending over backward to make sure he understood that this was in no way an ultimatum. The core of the story—that you asked the president for a raise—is true. But the way you tell the story is changed to make yourself look more forceful, bold, decisive—all of those traits you wish you had.

In riskier human interactions, lying *is* the right thing to do. "If Nazis are banging on your door asking for Anne Frank—and you know where she is—that's not the time to practice rigorous honesty," Lichtman says.

But if we wink at altruistic lies, overlook exaggerations, and nod with understanding at lies told to

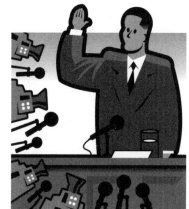

protect people from harm, we seem to have less ability to distinguish dishonesty used to manipulate, control, or make us look good. In an article that detailed one of the most comprehensive studies on lying ever conducted, Dr. DePaulo and her co-author found that the people who told more lies were "more manipulative, more concerned with self-presentation, and more sociable.... What is impressive about these people is that at the same time they are telling self-serving lies and getting their way, they still manage to be admired and even liked." (For more on how to spot a liar, see "The Lying Game" on page 54.)

Regardless of whether anyone catches on, such actions can be linked to several behavioral problems. Some people who tell lies simply refuse to take responsibility for their actions, says Glenda Wilkes, Ph.D., education professor in the department of educational psychology at the University of Arizona in Tucson. And if you won't take responsibility, you lie. "If you're constantly blaming your parents, your teachers, your boss, the environment, whatever, then you're less likely to be truthful," Dr. Wilkes says.

Others get in the habit of lying as a direct result of pressure to achieve placed on them by their parents, says C. R. Snyder, Ph.D., professor and director of the clinical psychology program at the University of Kansas in Lawrence. "This person could have had the fundamental dilemma from fairly early on that they weren't measuring up," Dr. Snyder says. "And I think one potential resolution of that is the lie. It becomes the little lie that becomes the big lie."

It's worth noting that excessive childhood lying is linked to more serious problems later on. "I found that children and adolescents who lie chronically—meaning enough over several

Nothing but the Truth

Not many of us would consider ourselves liars. But with the exception of when we're on the witness stand in a court of law, there aren't many of us who vow each day to "tell the truth, the whole truth, and nothing but the truth." Yet, that's precisely what Brad Blanton, Ph.D., author of *Radical Honesty*, thinks we should do.

Dr. Blanton believes that lying is the prime source of stress in our lives and that it's responsible for everything from physical and psychosomatic illnesses to the sky-high divorce rate. The answer, he says, is to always tell the truth to those closest to you—your family, friends, and co-workers.

If you're wondering what life would be like without those little white lies that get you through the day ("No, that dress doesn't make you look fat. You look great."), Dr. Blanton offers this suggestion: "Basically, I recommend that you find one other person and make an agreement for a definite period of time, for a month to six weeks, to just tell the truth about everything and see how it works. I recommend that you hurt people's feelings, but that you not just offend them and run off—that you stay with them. It doesn't take people more than 10 to 15 minutes to get over most hurt feelings and most anger. We can be furious at each other at 8:00, and by 8:15, we can go out and have a beer and be good friends."

months that it comes to the attention of teachers, friends, and family—have three times as many arrests as adults than those who don't lie frequently," says Paul Ekman, Ph.D., director of the Human Interaction Lab at the University of California Medical School in San Francisco and author of *Telling Lies*.

Truth or Consequences

There is another emotional problem that can trip you: Some guys never seem to grow out of their natural childhood fear of consequences, Dr. Wilkes says. When most kids get in trouble, they're more concerned about beating the rap than telling the truth. At about age 12, however, we're supposed to start shifting into a different mode. All of a sudden, you start doing good, moral things like sharing your lunch, picking on other kids less, and, low and behold, confessing youthful sins.

"By this point, kids really begin to have an understanding of honesty as a part of morality," Dr. Wilkes says. "Truth becomes important, and it's the morally correct thing to do. You have enough self-respect to not only see whether you're living an honest life but also to hold yourself accountable if you're not."

Dr. DePaulo and her co-author found that those study participants who told fewer total lies—especially self-serving lies—exhibited more of the traits that most men would want used to describe themselves: "responsible, honest, dependable, incorruptible, scrupulous, conscientious, reliable, stable, and straightforward." And in another victory for honesty, people who described their relationships with friends of the same gender as warm, enduring, and satisfying told fewer lies overall—and fewer self-centered lies.

Eventually, a few of us—like Mahatma Gandhi and the Rev. Dr. Martin Luther King, Jr.—reach the pinnacle: honesty in action—which is really another name for integrity, says Dr. Wilkes. "This is the point where some sort of greater good becomes more important." These people are willing to break a civil law, which is a form of dishonesty, for a greater good, such as the freedom of a people. And we

The Lying Game

Truth serums, lie detectors, even sharp sticks can all help you discover whether someone is being honest. But there are other ways to detect deception, according to the University of California Medical School's Dr. Paul Ekman.

After discovering what he believes are several universal clues to deceit, Dr. Ekman has spent the last two decades teaching members of the CIA, FBI, Drug Enforcement Administration, and Secret Service the tricks of the lying trade. Here's how to tell the truth.

Forget "false tells." You may have heard that someone is lying if they're doing things like pulling on their ears, rubbing their fingers, or looking away when they're talking. Or maybe their voice seems to go up an octave. In fact, these behaviors—which Dr. Ekman calls false tells—"could be due to a truthful person's fear of not being believed. I call this the Othello error after the Shakespearian character who didn't believe his wife Desdemona's denial of

all know how much respect men like that rightfully receive.

If you aspire to a more honest life, our experts recommend the following steps.

Consider the consequences. Your conscience may be asleep, but justice—like rust—never rests. "From all the lying I've examined, I've found that most lies eventually get discovered," Dr. Ekman warns. So before you tell that next lie, ask yourself: Is it truly worth risking my marriage, relationship, job, finances, or health? "One of the things I've found helpful with some of my students is to stop and examine yourself every time that you are about to tell something that is not true," Dr. Wilkes says. "Why am I going to say this?"

Think of the future. From a purely pragmatic standpoint, lying is not your best option. The problem with a lie is that, once told, it having an affair. Othello's error cost a lot of lives."

Pay attention to pauses. **Some people just speak slowly. But when they hesitate before answering a question that they shouldn't have to think about—like, "What did you do last night?"—you may be about to hear a lie, says Dr. Ekman.**

Indentify discrepancies. **Studying their face or voice or body language alone won't tell you whether someone is lying. Instead "look for discrepancies among all of them—when the speech doesn't match the facial expression, when the body language doesn't fit the voice," Dr. Ekman says.**

Keep them talking. **When the stakes are high, emotions can really help give liars away. But you have to keep them talking if you want the truth to come out. "Ask lots of open-ended questions and study their responses.... When the liar has shared values with the target of the lie, then the liar feels guilty about pulling off the lie," Dr. Ekman says.**

that sound suspiciously like someone who hasn't yet come to terms with who he is? Someone who needs outside approval? In other words, someone with a serious lack of self-respect? Remember: If you can't respect yourself, you can't expect others to respect you. (For more on self-respect, see page 38.)

Speak up. Failing to disclose important information isn't a lie, but it's still dishonest, Lichtman says. "Honesty and ethics are not about legal compliance," he says. "We can all think about times when the law fits one area, one narrow band, and then people have gone beyond it to take advantage of other people...even though they have been within the law. The question is, would you like to be treated like that?"

Quit the country club. People are inclined to lie when they're around people who don't appreciate them for who they are. So if Biff and Muffy have a nasty habit of making you feel like one of the hired hands, consider spending your time with a more encouraging group of friends. "You're looking for positive relationships, where other people aren't putting you down and they are appreciating your strengths," Dr. Snyder says. "That way you don't feel like you have to put on an act."

must be remembered forever. Otherwise, you may contradict yourself and expose yourself as a liar. The truth is easier to remember—after all, it's what really happened—and that makes it much easier to live with.

Look for patterns. If any of this sounds remotely familiar—and it might because we're all capable of such behavior—spend some time thinking about it. "You may not be dishonest in all phases of your life; you may only be dishonest with your girlfriend or your father or with your co-workers," Dr. Wilkes says. "If you can identify the pattern, where the problem areas are for you, then you have a better chance of changing that pattern. You can discover when it's going to come up."

Recommit to self-respect. Lots of guys lie to make themselves look better to the boss, to the ladies, to their buddies. But doesn't

Seek help and support. To say the least, most religions take a dim view of lying. ("A false witness will not go unpunished, and he who tells lies will perish." Proverbs 19:9) If you're having trouble with dishonesty, you might consider seeking spiritual counseling from a priest, minister, rabbi, or other religious leader, or joining a house of worship.

If you're not interested in a religious perspective, consider seeing a psychologist, Dr. Wilkes says. "It sounds like a cliché, but sometimes dealing with an issue like this is easier when you have someone there to help you through it," she says.

Humility

How to Be Strong—Nicely

It's one of the greatest sleight-of-hand tricks since David Copperfield bagged Claudia Schiffer: how to be assertive without being overbearing. To be confident without coming off as a braggart. To wield power and influence without being feared or distrusted.

The answer is a dose of old-fashioned humility. In this era of hotdogging, showboating, and other forms of shameless self-promotion, humility demonstrates a graciousness and depth and strength of character that can't help but command respect.

"To me, this is someone who feels no need to pretend, to posture and put on airs," says Dr. Michael Nichols of the College of William and Mary. "But (they) wouldn't necessarily come across looking meek. Rather, it would be someone who is calm and matter-of-fact about being who they are, with a fairly high degree of self-respect."

The Ways of Humility

Why do people brag? Often, to fulfill an emotional deficit that developed in childhood, experts say. "To the extent that you don't get admiring appreciation as a child, you always hunger for it...and some people show that hunger in rather obvious ways, like strutting and bragging and overachieving. It feels good, but it keeps us going on the treadmill of having to exaggerate, be terrific rather than being admired and appreciated and accepted for just being calmly and simply who we are," says Dr. Nichols. Here,

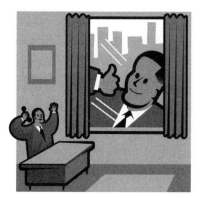

then, are ways to stay on the humble train.

Bag the rating game. If life were one endless talent competition, some of us might need to worry. Thankfully, it's not. The point being that you don't have to brag because, aside from yourself, no one on Earth is keeping score of your performance. Instead of comparing yourself to everyone else, learn to appreciate who you are. "If you were conceited and bragging all the time, but are now trying to achieve a certain amount of humility, you might say, 'Look, I am better looking. But that doesn't make me any better as a human being. Nor does it make me any worse if I'm not. I'm me and that's that,'" says Paul Hauck, Ph.D., a psychologist in Rock Island, Illinois, and author of *Overcoming the Rating Game.*

Lose the "me." It's the Golden Rule of dating, but it applies to virtually all conversations: To make a good impression, stop talking about yourself so much. Ask questions instead. Probe other people's ideas. It's so simple. How can you be humble if all you talk about is yourself?

Share the glory, accept the blame. The deal is signed, the game won, the good guys have emerged on top, and you are getting the credit. Your first action? No, don't go to Disneyland. Instead, spread the praise and glory all around. Tell those above and below you that you were just a small player in the success and that the success was due to everyone working together. Why? First, it's probably true, and even if not, it makes a big statement about what you are and aren't. But when things go bad, do the opposite: Own up to the mistake, take responsibility for the situation, and work to fix it. Don't grovel doing this—hold your head up, accept the heat, and learn from it.

Acknowledge being taught. People like nothing more than hearing that they have taught you something valuable. So express your appreciation when someone shares what they know with you, whether it is a specific job skill, a broad life lesson, or merely how to pronounce a word. After all, it takes humility to acknowledge to the world that everyone has things to teach you.

Assertiveness Made Easy

We're going to get right to the point here, fellas: One hallmark of healthy humility is getting right to the point—also known as assertiveness. "Assertiveness is about how to disagree without being disagreeable," says Sharon Anthony Bower, president of Confidence Training, based in Stanford, California, and co-author of *Asserting Yourself.* "It's a set of skills, communications skills, word skills, if you will, that help you get at the problem, not the person. It's important not to make people angry or afraid of you. That aggressive style does not encourage cooperation or respect."

We all seem to know that. Yet why do some us have such a hard time living it? "Often the men who have trouble with this were brought up in families where they were seen and not heard. They were brought up in a way that said, 'Don't ever question me.' And so they carry that misconception into life and into the workplace. They feel that if they don't say anything to others about their misgivings, then they are being respectful, because that's how they were brought up," says Bower. "In many cases, however, silence is not golden."

For those guys who are able to master true healthy assertiveness, increased respect for themselves and others awaits. "I think you gain respect for yourself when others can see that you want to control your anger. This gives you enormous power within a group or within a company. People can see that you're clear in what you say; you're objective. People feel safe with you. Every really respected leader gains power by being objective and clear," says Bower.

Learning how to communicate assertively takes time and education, and certainly Bower's book, co-written with her husband, Gordon H. Bower, Ph.D., a cognitive psychologist at Stanford University, is a good place to start. But here are some ways to start becoming more assertive now, according to Bower.

Be disagreeable—mildly. Ever see those wobbly-headed dogs that people put in the backs of their cars? Every time the car takes a bump in the road, the dog nods like the world is a giant Milk-Bone. Men who lack assertiveness may not be that compliant, but even when they disagree, they often remain silent just "for the sake of keeping the peace," says Bower. "It's okay to let people know that you disagree. Be direct. Simply say, 'I'm uncomfortable with that topic. I would rather talk about something else.' "

Seek clarity. No big secret. Real men hate to ask for directions when they're driving. But if someone gives you directions that you don't understand and you don't ask for clarification, that could also mean that you have a problem asserting yourself. "Rather than going away confused and feeling dumb, you can say, "I didn't understand your directions. Would you please go over them again?" says Bower.

Pull a Bob Marley. We're not talking about wearing dreadlocks, mon. But a persistent theme in reggae music—aside from the merits of ganja—is standing up for your rights. "Not allowing others to take advantage of you often requires standing up for your rights even though you may not always feel comfortable. You can learn to say no without feeling guilty. You can request your rights and ask to be respected. You can say, "I was next in line." Or, "Excuse me, I have another appointment now and must ask you to leave," Bower says.

Drive on. "If you have a legitimate complaint, you can continue to restate it until you get satisfaction, despite resistance from the other party. You should not allow a no to cause you to give up," says Bower.

Humor

Winning Respect with Your Wit

Let's face it: Your typical high-powered, chief executive officer would never be confused with Robin Williams. Yet even these stuffed shirts understand the value of a good yuk. A study of 737 of them found that 98 percent would rather hire somebody with a healthy sense of humor than one without.

If the poobahs in the corporate penthouse finally appreciate a joke or two—our salaries being the biggest joke of all—maybe it's because they're learning how hard the funny business can be. "Fear of public speaking is ranked number one on the list of fears in *The Book of Lists* and on most lists of what people are afraid to do," says Joel Goodman, Ed.D., director of The HUMOR Project in Saratoga Springs, New York, and co-author of *Chicken Soup for the Laughing Soul.* "I would probably say that there's a topper to that, and that's the fear of doing comedy in public. People appreciate people who are able to not only take the risk but also pull it off."

And when it works, though your life may not show it yet, you gain some personal power as well. "Some people think it's kid stuff, that it's not for keeps," says Dr. Goodman. "The reality is, if you take a look at the power of humor, it's a wonderful way of capturing attention, of having a group figuratively in the palm of your hand. And that's power. That's gaining control."

A well-timed joke or witty remark also does a great job of showcasing that awesome brainpower of yours—another respect-builder. Not sure how?

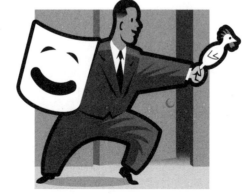

Consider this joke offered by Roger Langley, dean of the Comedy College in Rockville, Maryland: A Zen Buddhist goes to a ballpark and says to a hot dog vendor, "Make me one with everything."

When it comes to workplace stress reduction, humor is in a league of its own. "With change proverbially accelerating around us, how do we keep our balance, how do we keep control? How do we keep perspective? How do we keep on going? Humor is one thing that helps us do all that," says Dr. Goodman. "The notion of being able to laugh at yourself shows you're in control. That even a stressful situation isn't going to get the best of you."

On the Laugh Track

Thankfully, you don't have to be named Jay, Dave, or Rodney to add humor to your life. "There are thousands of ways of inviting smiles," says Dr. Goodman. Here's how it's done.

Get some attitude. Commanding respect isn't about issuing orders or looking stern. It's about being an ordinary guy and doing your best to exhibit some extraordinary character traits—among them the ability to laugh. But you never, ever want to take yourself too seriously. "Before you can start to develop your sense of humor, you have to have an attitude that says, 'Yeah, it's worth it. It's good for me. I need to be intentional about it.' So that certainly would be step one, just being aware that it's even possible to develop and use humor," says Dr. Goodman.

Have a vision. Maybe you like to laugh as much as the next guy but are concerned that you lack that all-important comedy performance gene. Thankfully, you won't have to wait for science to deliver. "Professional comedians look at the same chunks of reality that we all experience, and they see a humorous angle because they've developed a comic vision," says Dr. Goodman. To be a comic visionary in your own mind—if not someone else's—call a mental time-out for 5 minutes a day and look for the humor in the world around you or the world within you, he says. One way: Wait, *Candid Camera*–style, for someone around you to do something goofy— and then enjoy, he says.

Build a bulletin board of yuks. Surrounding yourself with wacky cartoons, silly faces, or cheap desk toys will almost certainly bring a smile to your face when life gets tough. "If you saw my office now, you would laugh. In fact, any photographer who shows up here just starts salivating. There's such an overload of stimuli. Funny photos...a caricature of me that was done a couple of years ago. It could be as simple as that," says Dr. Goodman. (By the way, it's now practically a federal law that your fridge door display at least one funny item. Don't make us turn you in.)

Grow some alligator skin. Unless you have your mommy on speed dial, whining about being the butt of a joke isn't going to cut it. Instead, develop a few snappy comebacks that will put any two-bit wisenheimer in his place. Or fire back with these oldies but goodies: "I resemble that remark" or "Oh yeah, you and what army?" says Dr. Goodman. They're stale as year-old rye, but sometimes you shouldn't look like you're trying too hard.

Create a running gag. Anytime something good happens to someone here at *Men's Health* Books, we pull out our trusty Nerf weapons and stage a sneak attack. Other folks get together to watch Must See TV. Whatever your preference, creating a running gag at your workplace or with your neighbors builds camaraderie and fun. "Those gags that have history and heritage don't require a set-up. Just the mere mention of the word or the calling up of the image or pulling out of the Nerf weapon, can, by itself, bring smiles and laughter to people," says Dr. Goodman.

Create a mirth-aid kit. Corny as it sounds, a basket full of funny videos and audiotapes, Slinkys, and action figures may just do the job during an IRS audit, plumbing problems, or at the first sign of a State of the Union address. "Sometimes you just need to give yourself a figurative shot in the arm," says Dr. Goodman.

Be careful with strangers. Giving the new vice-president a hard time about his lifetime membership to Hair Club for Men may seem like fun—until he arranges for you and your entire division to be transferred to Fargo, North Dakota. "You shouldn't tease total strangers. Sometimes you have no inkling of the way something is going to go over, whether it's going to hurt the person's feelings," says Robin Kowalski, Ph.D., associate professor of psychology at Western Carolina University in Cullowhee, North Carolina. "The risk is too great."

Watch it with women. Go a little easier on the gals since research shows they aren't into harsher forms of teasing. Then there's the issue of sexual harassment—two words which are never respectful or funny. Yet you face being accused any time you make a woman uncomfortable with your jests, no matter how tame or nonsexual you perceive your comments to be. "We did a narrative study where people wrote two stories: One about when they teased someone else and one about when they were teased, and the overall tone of the guys' stories was far more cruel than those written by the women," says Dr. Kowalski.

Also, watch the conclusions you draw when a female takes part in joking around. For example, the mere fact that a woman is teasing you does not mean she is flirting, says Dr. Kowalski. In fact, she probably isn't, and very well could be uncomfortable with the whole situation, but merely doing what she thinks she must to get ahead in a male-dominated office. Finally, always remember that what you find funny often is different from what she finds funny. Special note to Three Stooges fans: This means you.

Integrity

Living a Life That Counts

Of all the men Gary Oliver, Ph.D., has counseled through the years, there's one he'll never forget.

"He was in his early sixties, had over 15,000 employees, and flew in his own Learjet," recalls Dr. Oliver, psychology professor at Denver Seminary in Colorado; clinical director of Southwest Counseling Associates in Littleton, Colorado; and author of *Real Men Have Feelings Too.* "We got talking about his marriage and family, and here is this powerful guy who could buy me 10,000 times over with tears in his eyes.

"He was successful in every sense of the word except that his marriage was falling apart and none of his kids wanted to be in the family business. In fact, one of his sons told him that he had helped pay for the business by not having a father. He was relationally bankrupt, and I think that's part of it. People are starting to recognize the bankruptcy—the moral bankruptcy, the interpersonal bankruptcy—that occurs without integrity."

A Working Definition

In a survey of *Men's Health* magazine readers, integrity ranked second only to honesty as the quality most respected in other men. Another study found that men admire other men who are "dependable, honest, and authentic, not phony."

So what exactly is integrity? It's living your life

by a strict moral or ethical code, realizing that there are certain things about yourself, about who you are, that are not subject to compromise, and doing what you know is right rather than what is merely expedient.

Or, as the French novelist Paul Bourget once wrote: "One must live the way one thinks, or end up thinking the way one has lived."

When it comes to integrity, Stephen L. Carter, J.D., the William Nelson Cromwell Professor of Law at Yale University, wrote the book. Really. It's called (what else?) *Integrity.*

"Integrity requires three steps," Dr. Carter says. "Discerning what is right and what is wrong; acting on what you have discerned, even at personal cost; and saying openly that you are acting on your understanding of right from wrong."

Like most brilliant ideas, it's a pretty simple concept: Figure out what's right, do it, and then let people know why you did it. But in Dr. Carter's view, it's the hub on which all morality turns. "I really believe that without a sense of integrity, the rest of morality is meaningless because integrity suggests not that we have principles but that we are willing to stand up for them even when we risk losing something. And if we don't stand up for them, we don't know if we really have principles at all," explains Dr. Carter.

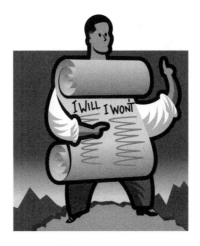

If you've found yourself drifting in a sea of questionable choices and shady dealings—at work as well as at home—it's time to shape up. Or as Dr. Carter quotes Thomas Aquinas: "Man has a natural aptitude toward virtue, but the perfection of virtue must be acquired through some aspect of training." Here's how to train for integrity.

Go deep. Job, entertainment, hobbies—a million things scream for our attention.

But until we take the time to look inward, we'll never know what we truly believe. "The first part, and a very hard one, is to be morally thoughtful," Dr. Carter says. "That is, when a person of integrity is faced with a difficult problem, he doesn't just say, 'Ha! I know the answer!' But he will instead spend the hard time to really try to do the work of discernment, perhaps to pray if he is religiously inclined, to find out what the answer is."

Start small. Once you've decided what's important, it's time to take action. "The second step is also a tough one. It is far easier to know what one believes—to know, in effect, right from wrong—than it is to do something about it," Dr. Carter says. "But we should start standing up for what we believe about little things. If there is an issue you're upset with a politician about, write a letter to the paper or the politician instead of just grumbling to your friends. Start with small things to exercise those virtue muscles. Suppose you really believe it's important to help the poor. Then you should be out there at the soup kitchens helping, instead of just voting for politicians who spend tax dollars on it."

Take a stand. By breaking your silence and letting others know what you're doing, you may encourage them to leave their comfort zone and pitch in. "I want to make it clear that I'm not talking about bragging, going around talking about what a great man of integrity I am," Dr. Carter says. "But the point is that a man of integrity is willing to stand by his principles, and that means that if he is challenged, he doesn't get mealymouthed.

"Suppose someone says, 'I don't like the way our government is spending our money,

---

Getting Carded

The Get Out of Jail, Free card has saved more than a few Monopoly players from a fictional hoosegow. But the folks at Texas Instruments have done them one better. For the past decade, the Dallas-based, high-tech giant has been giving new employees a wallet-size card that can help even the ethically impaired to do the right thing in virtually any situation. On one side the card reads:

- Is the action *legal*?
- Does it comply with our *values*?
- If you do it, will you feel *bad*?
- How will it look in the *newspaper*?
- If you know it's *wrong*, don't do it!
- If you're not sure, *ask*.
- Keep asking until you get an *answer*.

On the back: Encouragement to call the company's ethics office (toll-free) for "ethics answers."

"Ethical conduct within any kind of a large corporation is a shared responsibility," says Carl Skooglund, the company's vice-president and director of ethics. "It's a responsibility of the organization to help people know what is right and guide them through the process. And it's an individual's responsibility to help make the right personal choice. That's sort of reflected in the way that we have structured the questions. One of the things that we tell them is that if you answer question one no, you can skip the rest. That's where we draw the line."

All 59,000 of the company's employees receive a copy of the card as well as an ethics handbook, he says.

---

and therefore I am not going to pay my taxes in protest.' And then he gets caught by the IRS and says, 'Damn, those taxes slipped my mind.' That is just being a weasel. So it's being able to stand up at those hard moments and say, 'Yes, this is why I did what I did.' It's part of standing up for what we believe."

Be a man of your word. Since integrity is the basis for trust, broken promises and unfulfilled commitments just won't do. The most obvious way to prevent this from happening is keeping your word. "It's so important for us to keep our promises," Dr. Oliver says. "When we say it, people have to be able to take it to the bank."

Less obvious, but perhaps as important to helping you keep your commitments, is getting organized. If you know that your schedule is booked, you're less likely to bite off more than you can chew. Just don't use this as an excuse to avoid taking action.

Join a gang. Not the Crips or the Bloods, of course, but a growing number of men are finding that they are better able to live with integrity when they are members of what are called accountability groups. "I think that idea of accountability is very important," Dr. Oliver says. "I know that the guys who are going to carry me to my grave are going to be the guys I walked with while I was living. We need each other. Even the Lone Ranger had Tonto."

Dr. Oliver's group gets together over breakfast or coffee about every three weeks for a few hours, and inevitably discussion turns to a set of tough questions they created for each other. A typical question: "Have all my financial dealings been filled with integrity?"

Learn the art of compromise. It's one thing to stand up for what is true and good and right; it's another to be so obstinate that no one cares. Take government, for example. "I think that a person of integrity, while standing

Who Was That Masked Man?

What can a hopelessly outdated radio character—and his faithful companion—teach us about integrity today? Plenty, says ethics specialist Jim Lichtman, author of *The Lone Ranger's Code of the West.* "I don't think anyone would argue that we have a need today for greater consciousness and commitment to ethical values in our lives. And the Lone Ranger and Tonto can show us how," Lichtman says.

Billed as "an action-packed adventure in values and ethics with the legendary champion of justice," *The Lone Ranger's Code of the West* is based on the actual standards and background material created for the original show. The result is a lively look at honesty, fairness, caring, respect, loyalty, tolerance, duty, and moral courage through the eyes of the masked man himself. "The basic message of the book is, let's look at our own personal code and make some changes where we can so we can all make better decisions on a daily basis," Lichtman says.

Consider, for example, how you might react if you

for principle, also has to recognize that politics have to accomplish something," says Dr. Carter. "You are not there just to make speeches and introduce legislation that is just going to disappear. The idea is to accomplish something, to make the country better somehow."

This concept doesn't just apply to politicians. It's every bit as true in that murky world of office politics, too. If you adopt an all-or-nothing attitude toward your agenda, you may consistently wind up with nothing. It's better, Dr. Carter says, to compromise a little to gain as much of your goal as possible. "You don't just say that I am going to take my marbles and go home. You say that I am going to fight for as much of this as I can get. I am going to craft it heard that the Lone Ranger located the stolen payroll from the Lucky Strike mine, but before he returned the cash, he deducted for expenses like silver bullets, health insurance, and food while tracking the bad guys. Not only that but he and Tonto took it upon themselves to tack on a 30 percent finder's fee—only to have the Lone Ranger shortchange Tonto on his cut. "When I told this story at my seminars and everyone connected with it, I knew I was on to something," Lichtman says.

There is even a three-step decision-making process based on the values of the character.

1. The Lone Ranger considers the interests and well-being of all likely to be affected by his actions.

2. He makes decisions characterized by the core ethical values of honesty, fairness, caring, respect, loyalty, tolerance, duty, and moral courage to do what needs to be done.

3. If it is clearly necessary to choose one ethical value over another, the Lone Ranger will do the thing that he sincerely believes to be best for society in the long run.

to meet as many objections as possible and still save the core," Dr. Carter says.

Make amends. The question isn't whether we're going to make mistakes and do things we wish we hadn't done. That's a given. The question is, what do we do when it happens? "Admitting error is tremendously important," Dr. Carter says. "But you have to do it right. There is a risk that you could admit error that doesn't do anything but harm other people. In the 12-step programs, one of the steps is to make amends for things that you have done in the past, but they are careful to say that you make amends as long as you do it without making it worse, without hurting people.

"That's one of the big problems I have with all these books and television shows where people are confessing all their personal problems. Aside from the fact that they show no sense of shame for doing things that are wrong, there is a sense that I am going to just talk about whatever I want and let the chips fall where they may. And that is not integrity. Integrity does certainly mean confessing an error, but only if you can do it in a way that isn't going to make things worse. It's not confession for its own sake."

Be a mensch. You don't have to be Jewish to know what a mensch is—or to use the word. And you certainly don't have to be Jewish to *be* a mensch. It comes from the Yiddish word *mensh*, meaning "human being," but it has come to mean "a person of integrity and honor."

Rabbi Harold Kushner, popular author of *When Bad Things Happen to Good People* and *How Good Do We Have to Be?*, adds to that definition: "...sensitivity and concern for others, a sense of responsibility, reliability, somebody you can trust, someone you admire. It's the Jewish version of human fulfillment or enlightenment. But it's a down-to-earth quality, a this-worldly sainthood. A Hassidic sage once said, 'God has enough angels; he needs more menschen.'"

In *The Joys of Yiddish*, novelist Leo Rosten writes: "It is hard to convey the special sense of respect, dignity, approbation, that can be conveyed by calling someone 'a real mensh.' As a child I often heard it said, 'The finest thing you can say about a man is that he is a mensh.' To be a mensh has nothing to do with success, wealth, status. The key...is nothing less than character: rectitude, dignity, a sense of what is right, responsible, decorous. Many a poor man, many an ignorant man, is a mensh."

So if you want to get some respect, be a mensch.

Trust

The Key to Winning Loyalty

A 90-year-old Lawrence, Massachusetts, textile mill—one of the last still operating in the Northeast—burns to the ground, throwing 3,000 people out of work two weeks before Christmas. The easiest thing for owner Aaron Feuerstein to do: collect the insurance money and retire. After all, the guy just turned 70.

Cashing in is the last thing on his mind. Feuerstein not only promises to rebuild but also continues to pay the salaries of his idled workers, extends their health benefits, even makes sure that each gets their annual Christmas bonus. A note he sends to each says simply, "Do not despair. God bless each of you." Within two months, 70 percent of his workforce is back on the job.

If the nation needed a poster boy for trustworthiness and loyalty, this feisty, proverb-spouting granddad was suddenly it. His self-assured, never-surrender expression graced newspapers around the country and magazines from *People Weekly* to *Forbes*. President Bill Clinton showed his appreciation by inviting Feuerstein to a State of the Union address. And even a few years later, those who write about business management and ethics still laud him as a hero and example of good and responsible corporate behavior. "Have you ever seen the statue of George Washington in New York City's financial district?" asks Wess Roberts, Ph.D., a psychologist and author of *Protect Your Achilles Heel* and *Leadership Secrets of Attila the Hun*. "I think they should put one of Aaron Feuerstein next to the statue of George—only it ought to be bigger. I really admire and respect the loyalty he and his

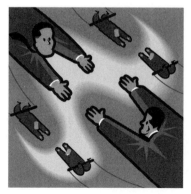

company showed their employees."

All that praise may seem excessive until you ponder how rare such trustworthy bosses—heck, husbands, brothers, friends—are these days. Forget the headlines that daily chronicle the collapse of trustworthiness. One study says it all: When folks were asked whether they thought most people could be trusted, researchers found that those saying yes plunged from 58 percent in 1960 to 37 percent in 1993.

Now if trust was just another pleasant rule of etiquette, that statistic might not have much relevance. But a growing number of experts react to these dwindling levels of loyalty with serious concern and dismay.

"The decline of trust and sociability...is also evident in...the rise of violent crime and civil litigation; the breakdown of the family structure; the decline of a wide range of intermediate social structures like neighborhoods, churches, unions, clubs, and charities; and the general sense among Americans of a lack of shared values and community with those around them," writes Francis Fukuyama, author of *Trust: The Social Virtues and the Creation of Prosperity*. "This decline of sociability has important implications for American democracy, perhaps even more so than for the economy."

We're already paying a direct tax imposed by the breakdown of trust in society in the form of ever-increasing police protection, a prison system far larger than any other industrialized country, and lawyers who earn substantially more than lawyers in Europe or Japan, so Americans can sue each other, contends Fukuyama.

Now, before you head to your local Army surplus store and start restocking your bomb shelter, consider a more positive alternative: If distrust and betrayal play a big role in these and other social problems, the opposite must be true—building trust and loyalty can help stem the decline. We can reduce lawlessness by telling the truth ourselves. Every promise kept—no matter how small—is another sturdy knot in the social fabric of the republic. Every handshake deal observed, a high five for truth, justice, and the American way. And if you're not exactly Mr. Patriotic? We not only help our nation but we also help ourselves.

"Credibility is not about looking good; it is about being good," writes Blaine Lee, Ph.D., founding vice-president of the Covey Leadership Center in Salt Lake City, in his book *The Power Principle: Influence with Honor.* "You can be unconditionally trustworthy. As you strive for such trustworthiness, your perceived credibility will increase."

The Hopeful Journey to Trust

But before we march together toward this brighter, more respectful, tomorrow, let's take a closer look at what trust is—and isn't. Dr. Lee puts it this way: "Trust is not blind faith, lemminglike followership, a suspension of the desire or ability to make independent assessments..., giving up deeply held values, dreams, or desires for the 'good of the organization.'" So much for all those company men who compromise first and ask questions later.

True trust is built on thoughtful promises made and kept. "When we make commitments to others, when we communicate intent, when we make promises and create expectations, the direct result is hope.... If the expectations we create are realized, and others learn about this, then we move beyond hope to trust," writes Dr. Lee.

From a promise to hope to trust. And the amazing thing is that this concept applies to virtually every human interaction: from taking your dog to the vet with the expectation that the doc has legitimate credentials, to believing that the guy who refs your night basketball league will truly call 'em as he sees 'em. Or in the case of Aaron Feuerstein, rebuilding his company just as he said.

And when trust is fulfilled, you don't just get your job back or a warm, fuzzy feeling. Something else magical happens: loyalty. "I

The Truth about Handshakes

We think nothing of clasping hands as a sign of friendship, respect, or even to seal a deal. But folklore tells us that it may have been a way to make sure the other guy wasn't packing some kind of weapon.

It seems that it was customary in some cultures for a man to draw his dagger when he came face-to-face with someone new. The two guys would circle each other until they were satisfied that the other guy wasn't going to attack, and then put their weapons away. The weapon-carrying hand was then extended "as a token of goodwill," says to Charles Panati, author of *Extraordinary Origins of Everyday Things*.

In ancient Egypt, it was thought the handshake conferred power from a god to an earthly ruler. Babylonian kings shook hands with a statue of their chief deity once a year, symbolizing a transfer of authority.

To shake it up the right, respectful way:

Make sure the webbing between your thumb and index finger meet his. Grasp his whole hand. Use firm pressure, but don't crush. You may respect someone who just broke several of your bones, but you won't trust him very much. Look the person in the eye as you give one full shake. Short, firm, confident.

trust you that when you tell me something, you're going to do it," says Dr. Kate Wachs of The Relationship Center. "You earn my loyalty when my trust has been confirmed."

If you're still having trouble seeing the connection between trust, loyalty, and respect, consider what a *Men's Health* magazine poll discovered. It found that loyalty was one of the five qualities that readers respect in other men. Among the five qualities named in the poll so heinous as to negate all of a man's good qualities: cheating and infidelity—trust-busters if we've ever seen them.

Building Trust

We won't kid you guys, building trust isn't always easy—nor the ways readily apparent. But there are several overarching approaches that, once learned, can boost trust from the family room to the workplace—and all points in between. Here's how to go about it. And when you need inspiration, it can't hurt to think of Aaron Feuerstein.

Check your roots. You've heard it in different ways elsewhere in this book, but it bears repeating: We all need to take time to reflect on our levels of trustworthiness and loyalty. For some guys, this may mean an extended time of self-evaluation, maybe even a sabbatical from the job. For others, it's shooting the breeze while eating breakfast once a week with some pals. In either case, you need to assess what kind of man you are, what kind of man you want to be, and what it will take to make the two match.

"Here's an analogy for you: People are like trees," says Denver Seminary's Dr. Gary Oliver. "The shadow of the tree is the reputation, the fruit of the tree is the personality, but the root system of the tree—the most important part—is the character. And eventually, the root system is going to affect the fruit and the shadow of the tree."

Create your own board of directors. Who would top your list of most trustworthy heroes. Mahatma Gandhi? Winston Churchill? Muhammad Ali? Billy Graham? Martin Luther King, Jr.? Pope John Paul II? Cal Ripken, Jr.? "Learn everything you can about them. Make these people your personal board of directors, and when you're faced with a moral dilemma, ask yourself what they would do," says Randy G. Pennington, president of Pennington Performance Group, a Dallas-based training and consulting firm, and author of *On My Honor, I Will: Leading with Integrity in Changing Times.*

Stop the small stuff. Trust is destroyed with one devastating blow—like sexual infidelity—but it's also eroded over time by breaking small, seemingly insignificant promises or saying things that we don't mean. "Don't say anything that you can't do, don't say anything that you don't mean," says Dr. Wachs. "You want to be responsible for what you say, like it's a mini-commitment. Don't be rude, but say what you mean and then act that way. Keep your actions and statements in sync."

Deliver the message. In the office, it's making sure that an employee doesn't hear at the watercooler that you're thinking about canceling his project. With a friend, it's telling him that you're thinking about dating his ex—rather than letting him hear it on the street. "You keep people informed about the vital issues, and in return, they're going to keep you informed. And that creates trust," says Dr. Roberts.

Give people a chance. Whether it's a dad angrily pulling a rake out of his son's hands, or a chief executive officer taking away your most lucrative account, hastily removing someone from a job is one of the quickest ways to show disrespect and lack of trust. Instead, try to appreciate the other person's strengths and gifts, and give them a chance to perform. They may not do it exactly the way you want it done, but they're probably doing the best they can. "It's about recognizing the expertise that they bring and trusting them to use it," says Dr. Roberts.

Throw a block. Sometimes, in football, all it takes is one well-timed block to spring even the slowest back on a touchdown run. In the same way, a dad or boss can help build trust by running interference for the people closest to him, says Dr. Roberts. "To the degree that you can, keep people out of their way who are trying to interfere with them doing their jobs, and keep the level of aggression and interference out of the workplace as much as you can," he says. "They'll learn that they can rely on you."

Train your troops. What's one of the first things that happens when you join the military—besides getting a buzz cut? Training, son, and lots of it. This builds trust from top to bottom because the soldiers know that the other guys in the trenches have been trained to do their job, says Dr. Roberts. In the same way, help your friends, co-workers, and employees get the training they need to develop themselves more fully, and watch your trust in them soar.

Bail not. Nothing destroys loyalty quicker than bailing on a buddy when he needs you most—especially if *you* caused the problem. "Accept complete responsibility for your actions, especially when it's convenient to blame others. Actively accepting responsibility forces us to evaluate the impact of our decisions prior to our actions," says Pennington.

When Trust Has Been Shattered

It's a painful rebuilding process, but trust can, and should, be restored. If not just for reasons of mutual respect, then for your health. "I've noticed that when people keep some kind of deep betrayal inside, they eventually develop all kinds of strange symptoms," says Dr. Wachs. "There's nothing medically wrong, but they start running fevers, throwing up, or the blood pressure goes up and they have a heart attack. You're not made to keep all that stress in." Here's how to get on the road to emotional—and physical—recovery when trust has been lost.

Face the music. Whether you're the guy who did the dirty deed or the one it has

been done to, stuffing your feelings and trying to forget is absolutely the wrong approach. "The first thing you have to do is talk about it," Dr. Wachs says. "Even if you don't see the person again, you have this lingering unresolved memory that comes crashing back every time something reminds you." If you feel like you can't talk to a good friend about it, join a therapy group or see a professional, she says.

Speak from the heart and learn. You're darn right you're mad. And well you should be—your trust has been trashed. So tell the person how you feel, using "I" statements. Not, "you make me so angry." But, "when you did that, I felt like I was going to explode." "Depending on the situation, you're going to have feelings of anger, betrayal, disappointment, embarrassment, and maybe some worry about whether you're man enough," says Dr. Wachs. "Making someone have this conversation won't allow them to just forget about it. Plus, you're more likely to get an apology. If they don't apologize and they don't get it straight in their mind, then it's more likely to happen again. The way people keep making the same mistake is that they just sort of shut it out of their consciousness."

Seek to understand. The last thing you want to hear are a bunch of lame excuses. But there might actually be something going on that you don't know about that contributed to the betrayal. "Maybe he has a drinking problem, maybe he has been taking drugs, maybe he's angry with you for something you did to him," says Dr. Wachs. "There are usually reasons that somebody tries to hurt you, and in a way, it's good to know that because it can make it feel a lot less personal."

Forgive. Yes, it's going to take time. And you may never be able to trust this guy again, but that's no reason to allow a grudge to literally take you to your grave. One way to do it if the guy isn't around: Visualize him in an empty chair across from you and pour out your anger. Or write a letter and tear it up—and with it your feelings of resentment.

Wisdom

Get Smart and Get Respect

With all due respect to that famous smart guy Albert Einstein, we just have to wonder how much common sense the great man had. As most of us know, Einstein developed the theory of relativity—whatever that is—and even nailed down a Nobel Prize in physics. Impressive stuff—especially for those of us who feel like we deserve a call from the Nobel committee just for being able to file our taxes.

But as it turns out, Mr. E=MC² was so often lost in deep, smart-guy thoughts that he would leave his home and wander down the street without first stopping to put on his shoes. "That, obviously, did not demonstrate what is conventionally known as wisdom," says Michael Jacobson, Ph.D., a professional educator based in Chicago and the director of science and education for MENSA, an organization for people with high IQs.

The point: If you're a genius (mathematical, comic, or otherwise), you may lack common sense and do rather well—as long as your feet are reasonably tough. And if you're a regular guy who wants to command respect like the rest of us? You'll need to develop a mixture of book smarts *and* common sense—in other words, wisdom.

You see, gents, it's like this: If intelligence is a measure of how much information you have tucked in your cranium, wisdom is the ability to use that information in a meaningful way—whether you're at the dinner table fielding tough questions from your kids or at the conference table divining a new marketing strategy. "A

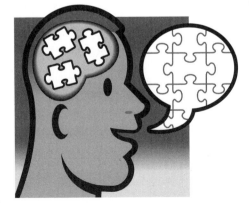

wise person is defined as someone who can take a problem and put it into perspective and who knows the proper ways of handling it," says Dr. Jacobson. Or as Thomas J. Watson, the man who dragged IBM into the early computer age, put it: "Wisdom is the power that enables us to use knowledge."

Wisdom of the Smart and Famous

If one grows wiser with age, as the saying goes, it is because with age comes experience. You have traveled more, been in more sticky situations, seen fads and presidents come and go, succeeded and failed more. And with all this experience, you learned what matters and what doesn't, and how to put the small events of daily life in their proper context.

A fuller view of true wisdom comes to us from Criswell Freeman, doctor of psychology and the author of *Wisdom Made in America* and *When Life Throws You a Curveball, Hit It.* After studying the lives of literally thousands of famous and important people, Dr. Freeman says he has noticed five characteristics that seem common to many. They are:

- *Perspective.* "Most of us are prisoners of the urgent rather than servants to the important. These people are able to step back. They view life as a landscape rather than a close-up. They say, 'This is a small problem that I don't even need to worry about.'"
  - *Purpose.* "By stepping back, they can then say, 'I may have 15, 30, 50 years left, and this is what I want to do with it.' They develop a sense of purpose...a mission."
  - *Proactivity.* "Talk is very cheap. Everyone says, 'I'm going to get around to it eventually.' But the fact is that these are

people who said they were going to do something and, by golly, they went and did it."

- *Persistence.* "It's rare that any important project is going to be a hit the first time out. You don't step up to the plate in an important ball game and expect that you are going to hit four home runs. The idea is that the really great minds continue to pursue, despite the inevitable failures."
- *Optimism.* "When was the last time that you saw a statue built to a pessimist? Without optimism, you look at the future and it's all kind of gray and dark and you say, 'What's the use?' With it, the future is boundless."

Cultivating Intelligence

Despite what you might think, the experts tell us there are only two ways to measure intelligence: testing what you know and testing your ability to solve word or mathematical problems. If you increase your level of general knowledge or sharpen your problem-solving ability, bingo, "you're going to score higher on those tests," says Dr. Jacobson.

But you'll do much more. "Ideally, every person who wants to command respect has to be reasonably informed and educated," says Kenneth C. Davis, author of the million-plus selling *Don't Know Much About...* series of books on history, geography, and the American Civil War. "A person who can sit at a corporate board meeting or a sales conference table and discuss with a degree of certainty and correctness historical events, facts, and dates and relate them to what's going on today is going to go far."

To build a broad body of knowledge, consider these tips.

Do some mental gymnastics.

Whether it's unraveling the mysteries the *New York Times* crossword puzzle or watching the Discovery Channel, take every opportunity you can to acquire more information. "You have to exercise those brain cells. In fact, studies are

starting to show that those who have above-average verbal intelligence and who frequently use their intellectual capability have a lower incidence of Alzheimer's disease," says Dr. Jacobson.

Be curious. It sounds like a contradiction, but having a childlike sense of wonder about the world around you is one of the surest paths to a mature wisdom. Probe the mysteries of the world around you. How do you make a microchip? What does sea urchin taste like? How did they build that bridge? What do Buddhists believe in? How do they put wax on cucumbers? The wisest people often have an insatiable hunger for knowledge. For them, it is a game, a pleasure, a reason for existing.

Tune in to Amadeus. It's no surprise that head-banging isn't so great for the brain. But listening to Mozart appears to be a different story. At least one study of college students found that those who listened to Mozart for 10 minutes before an IQ test scored better than those who listened to a relaxation tape or nothing at all. Researchers suspect that Mozart's classical yet complex sounds may somehow stimulate brain activity.

Declare your dependence. If you're a brooding loner, you may be the next James Dean, but at least one study shows that you're not nearly as smart as you could be. The study found that guys who feel comfortable asking questions and who look to others for guidance had high school grade point averages in the 3.0 to 3.25 range. Those who prefer to tackle tasks on their own, on the other hand, had averages in the 2.8 to 3.0 range. The bottom line is that asking more questions may make you smarter.

Do some fiddling. Whether it's taking up the violin or trying to fix a broken toaster, research shows that challenging new activities can stimulate your brain in a way that probably adds to its computational power. The trick is to try something different from what you do by day—something Einstein apparently knew since he played the violin.

Master your memory. Nothing can make you look like an absent-minded professor quicker than poor recall. But building an impressive short-term memory ain't rocket science—all you need is a little concentration and imagination. For example, when you meet someone and they tell you their name, simply repeat it out loud and then associate it with something unusual or unique about them. Let's say you just shook hands with lovely Carmen. Imagine Carmen driving a huge car that was being chased by thousands of men. Or if she wasn't quite so lovely, you could imagine a very large Carmen chasing after you as you drive away. If leaving stuff behind (à la Einstein) is your problem, park the items in question in a prominent place near the front of the door so you can't miss them. To keep track of shades, keys, and other easy-to-lose personal items, create a home for them and put them there as soon as you enter your dwelling.

Develop some healthy habits. On the way home from the library or bookstore (or Carmen's), don't forget to stop at the gym. Regular exercise—as in 30 minutes a day, at least three times a week—has been found to reduce your risk for cardiovascular disease. How does that help upstairs? The muscle-building effect that keeps your heart healthy in turn makes sure it's pumping the proper amount of blood to your brain—mandatory for intelligent thinking. Ditto for getting at least the Daily Value for vitamins such as C, B_{12}, E, thiamin, riboflavin, and niacin and the minerals boron and zinc. Research also shows some benefit on brain function from nutritional supplements such as ginkgo biloba and lecithin. Use as directed.

Further Lessons in Wisdom

Whether you're already a graduate of the school of hard knocks, a new student, or somewhere in between, there are some things that you can do to help you get yourself wiser, faster. Here's how it's done.

Try some fables. You could spend hours trying to wade through Plato's *Republic* or the convoluted logic of Aristotle. But if you really want to learn basic philosophy without putting yourself into a coma, check out *Aesop's Fables*. Thought to be written by a Greek slave, these short, easy-to-read tales teach moral lessons that are still applicable today. The best example: *Aesop's The Hare and the Tortoise.* "These teach life skills, problem solving...they are the greatest primers on ethics and philosophy that I've ever read," says Dr. Jacobson.

Spend some time with Dad. Remember him? The guy who wiped your butt and was also named most respected in a poll of *Men's Health* magazine readers should be a veritable font of wisdom at this stage of life. "We need to take advantage of the knowledge that our parents and grandparents have," says Dr. Jacobson. "They possess the wisdom of having walked in your shoes before you even owned shoes. This is a true crash course in wisdom." The next best thing: fishing with a guy Dad's age. (For more on the benefits of spending time with Dad, see The Virtuous Son on page 94.)

Develop your emotional intelligence. Since no one seems wiser than the person who is able to control his emotions, it would probably be smart to develop what's called your emotional intelligence. "The first step is to recognize that an emotion is being triggered, instead of being caught in a state in which all you are thinking is, 'I hate you, you S.O.B.,' " says Daniel Goleman, Ph.D., a behavioral sciences writer for the *New York Times* and author of *Emotional Intelligence.* "If you can stop yourself and simply say, 'Oh, I'm angry,' you are beginning to practice a kind of self-reflection called mindfulness. Just by activating this self-reflexive awareness, you're triggering areas of the brain that actually short-circuit the reactive emotional centers. This...opens the door to the other ways to prevent emotional hijacking: managing anger and handling anxiety, the ability to motivate yourself through hopefulness, empathy, and developing the kinds of social skills that enable people to feel good about your interactions with them."

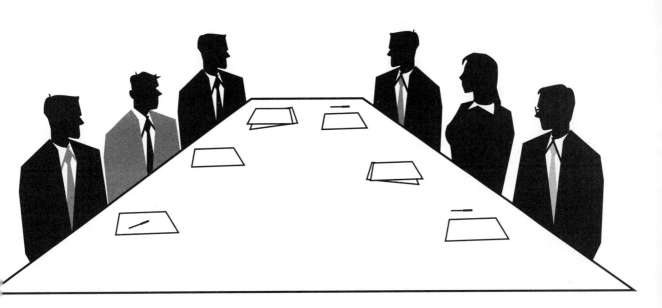

Part Three

Working on Respect

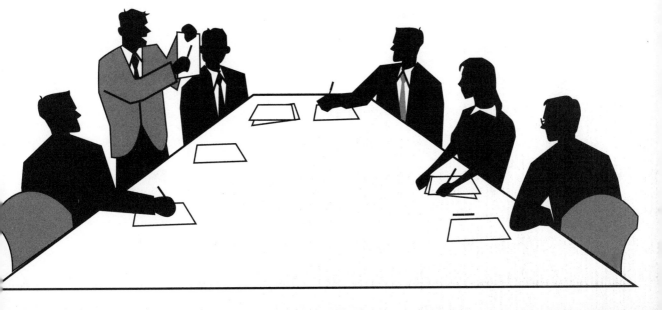

Give Respect, Get Results

Timeless Wisdom Takes Hold in the Business World

What does it mean when one of the most popular cartoons in America, Dilbert, spends each day detailing the hardships of an employee forced to work in an "incredible shrinking cubicle" and deal with a boss who threatens to fire the staff and replace them with "easily trainable native Eskimos?" Or perhaps, worst of all, that the material is based on actual workplace events sent to the cartoonist from working people around the country?

Sad to say, too many workplaces lack respect. But a growing number of experts believe that the path to improving job performance is a simple matter of treating others with time-honored principles like honor and respect. And for bosses and companies weary of trying to solve core business problems with management fad-of-the-month solutions, the concept is suddenly ringing true.

"True lasting power doesn't flow from titles or tactics, persuasion, or intimidation," says Blaine Lee, Ph.D., founding vice-president of the Covey Leadership Center in Salt Lake City and author of *The Power Principle: Influence with Honor.* "Principle-centered leaders understand that the principles you lead your organization by create your culture. If I honor and respect you and you, in turn, feel honor for me, some remarkable things are possible."

"You can do this without any input from top management," points out Stephen J. Holoviak, former director of the

Frehn Center for Management at Shippensburg University in Pennsylvania and author of *Golden Rule Management: Give Respect, Get Results.* "Treating people with respect and dignity shouldn't be against any company policy."

Casting Off Old Patterns

Whenever people come together in groups, they tend to recreate the emotional dynamics of families, says Brian DesRoches, Ph.D., a Seattle-based therapist and author of *Your Boss Is Not Your Mother.* Is it any wonder, then, that trouble at work makes us feel like we're "kids relating to overbearing fathers, guilt-tripping mothers, teasing older brothers, and competitive sisters?" he asks.

The problem is that we often react as we did in family situations—complaining, accusing, internalizing, rebelling. Does any of that sound like smart business practice? Here, then, are ways to give and get respect in the workplace the professional way.

Can the coercion. Attila the Boss is an intriguing office fantasy—imagining yourself wearing a menacing-looking helmet with wings on it, waving your sword at slow-moving employees—but coercive behavior often spells doom. Not so much for those whom you threaten, but for yourself. "Sometimes the result of coercing people is the illusion of control that comes short-term," says Dr. Lee. "If you threaten someone long enough, they are going to respond, but when you are gone, what

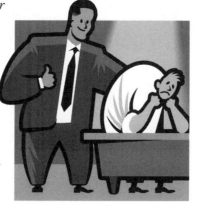

happens? Maybe some people would say, 'We won't get mad, we'll get even.' And so sabotage is the result. The result of fear is always negative."

Don't fake power. Some guys pretend that they have power even when they don't. And most often, they do this by being rude. "Rudeness...will get me the seat in the restaurant I want.

Just kind of bully my way in. (But) rudeness is the insecure person's imitation of power. It's a pretense," says Dr. Lee.

End the blame game. One of the first skills we learn as kids—aside from drawing on the freshly painted walls of our rooms—is to blame others. In the work world, blaming others for mistakes or failures—things like, "I haven't gotten a raise because my boss is a jerk," or "I didn't meet my deadline because the place is a sweatshop"—not only is unprofessional and hostile but also is a formula for corporate failure. Instead, try to apply no-fault thinking, says Dr. DesRoches. "No-fault thinking means saying no one is to blame but everyone is responsible. I am responsible. And so is everyone else. What is my responsibility? That focuses attention on yourself, where the change can happen, and where you can really make a difference. This is the most important thing to remember, yet it's the most difficult."

Ask rather than react. If Mr. Spacely blasts your design for a new sprocket by calling you a dope, pause and ask him to tell you more—rather than reacting in anger. "When people make statements like that, obviously there isn't any thinking going on. It's a totally emotional statement and a reaction. He is probably threatened or feels incompetent," says Dr. DesRoches. Asking for more information shows that you're still under control and forces the other person to think over what they are saying—and that could lead to a calmer, more thoughtful response from them, he says.

Learn to count. When you're beginning to stress out, your body sends you all kinds of clues: Your palms sweat, your heart races, your colon does the macarena. It's in these moments that we can really lose respect—for ourselves and others. "I'm recommending that you

Childish Roles

It's pretty obvious that the way we interact with others was shaped by our relationships with our parents and siblings as we grew up. But what's less obvious is how we take those social patterns and apply them in our adult life, particularly at work, says therapist Dr. Brian DesRoches, author of *Your Boss Is Not Your Mother*.

There are at least four roles developed in the home that guys play on the job that can prevent them from getting—or giving—respect, according to Dr. DesRoches.

- The Rebel. **The black sheep of the family, this is the guy who learned to get attention by causing trouble and hanging with the bad boys. At work, he'll lead "uprisings," quit his job in a huff, or force the boss to fire him.**
- The Victim. **A child of overbearing parents, victims put their jobs first and their needs second. They go out of their way to avoid conflict and are insecure.**
- The Rescuer. **This guy may seem like he's being altruistic by helping other people, but it could just be his way of avoiding his own problems. Just as his brothers and sisters came to him for advice and comfort, he gets his attention by being kind and caring.**
- The Persecutor. **Bosses and back-stabbing colleagues aren't the only ones who appear to play this role. Saying no or refusing to get involved in office shenanigans can also get you labeled as a persecutor.**

become an expert at observing your own emotional process. What happens in your body when you get reactive? The old adage about counting to 10 is great wisdom. Great wisdom. Grandma was right." And then proceed with caution, says Dr. DesRoches. "You can't talk yourself out of problems that you've behaved yourself into," Dr. Lee says.

On the Job Interview

Pursuing Hire Education

It was just another job interview for a senior marketing position when a lack of respect —and common sense—reared its ugly head.

"The client and I were interviewing the gentleman and in the midst of our discussion, a beeper started going off," says Jude Werra, owner and president of Werra and Associates, an executive search firm in Brookfield, Wisconsin. "He reached into his breast pocket and pulled out some kind of little contraption. And we said, 'What's that?' And he said, 'I'm quitting smoking and this time is when I can have a cigarette. So I have to go have a cigarette now. If I don't, my smoking-cessation program will be out of whack.' And with that, he excused himself and went out to have a cigarette."

Obviously, the guy's job opportunity also went up in smoke. But while interview blunders of this magnitude may be rare, there are dozens of small ways you can tank your chances. "I've had recruiters tell me they make their decision within the first couple of minutes. And then the rest of the interview is justifying it," says Barbara Pachter, president of Pachter and Associates in Cherry Hill, New Jersey, and co-author of the *Prentice Hall Complete Business Etiquette Handbook*. "It's that old adage: You never get a second chance to make a first impression."

Earning Respect— And a Paycheck

If the impression you make on prospective employers is one of the utmost respect for yourself and others, you're bound to get hired, says Richard Bolles, author of *What Color Is Your Parachute?* "In this age of rudeness, lies, manipulation, and getting ahead at any cost, you will want, above all else, to be a beacon of integrity, truth, and kindness throughout your job hunt or career change.... *That's* the kind of employee employers are dying to find."

Consider these tips as you set out on your job search.

Set a goal. Even before you pick up the classifieds or phone that headhunter your buddy told you about, set a goal for your job search. "Say to yourself, 'I'm going to make 10 contacts a week; I'm going to send out this many résumés.' You set the number, but make it realistic, and that will keep you focused," Pachter says.

Prepare for the Big Five. Rather than memorizing snappy answers to millions of job-related questions, Bolles says the person who can hire you will basically want to know five things: "Why are you here? What can you do for us? What kind of person are you? What distinguishes you from the 19 other people who can do the same tasks that you can? And can I afford you?" Since these questions form the backbone of most interviews, if you're able to answer these, chances are good that you'll be able to field anything else they throw at you, he says.

Get a Jimmy Johnson. Not his hairstyle, tough guy—but someone you can report to every week to make sure that you're sending out those résumés and going on those interviews. "I call this person a job coach," Pachter says. "They should keep you accountable in terms of how many places you're going to apply, etcetera."

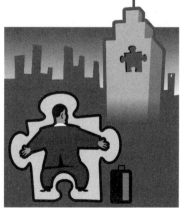

Suit up. What with the trend toward casual office-wear, fewer guys are wearing suits and ties. But if you ever needed to be a sharply dressed man, your interview is it. "You may not feel like you need a new suit, but when you're doing job interviews, I think you should go out and buy one you can afford," Pachter says. "You're going to get a lot of wear out of it. As long as it's clean and pressed, you can wear it to a lot of different interviews." And when you land the crucial follow-up interview? You have two choices: Buy another one or wear another one—you don't want to show up in the same outfit—yet.

Bring a briefcase. Brown paper bags work for hoagies, plastic for the trash, even Styrofoam for brew, but you need an attractive briefcase or satchel to tote your flawless résumé, notepad, attractive pen, and other job search–related items. And don't ever put it down on the interviewer's desk. "It sounds dumb, but people do it," Pachter says.

Exchange pleasantries. After looking the job interviewer in the eye and applying a firm handshake (grip the web of the palm, please), a standard, "Good morning/afternoon/evening, it's nice to meet you" is basic and fine. From there, it might be a good idea to have a "pleasant self-revelation" planned, says Pachter. "Not 'I ran over a cat on my way here.' But something like, 'It has been a wonderful trip to New York; I just got to see my college roommate whom I haven't seen in years.' I did this during one of my interviews and all of a sudden we're on to a real happy conversation about where we went to school, and colleges, and reunions. And I got the job." Coincidence? We think not. And by the way, it's okay to use the same pleasantry for other interviews.

Do a time check. Before the ball gets rolling, find out how much time you have for the interview. "Lots of people forget to ask and wait until later to ask their questions, but time runs out and they never get to ask them," Werra points out.

Take some notes. Before the heavy-duty discussion begins, suavely reach into your briefcase and pull out your handy notepad and pen and commence note taking. How much? You shouldn't scribble so furiously that the interviewer becomes acquainted with the top of your head, but enough so that you will be able to ask some good questions later. "You don't want it to become a distraction for them or you," Pachter says. "But there's a proverb: 'The palest ink is better than the best memory.'"

Pay later. "In lots and lots of interviews these days, salary is negotiable—if you save the discussion to the very end of the interviewing process," Bolles says. His advice: Never be the first to mention salary; decide before you interview how much you really need, factoring in benefits; research pay ranges in your field and for that organization, and then when they say they can't live without you and make an offer, take your best shot. "I understand, of course, the constraints under which all organizations are operating in the 1990s, but I believe my productivity is such that it would justify a salary in the range of... and here you mention the figure near the top of their range," Bolles says. Be prepared to say how you will make or save the company money, and get your salary agreement in writing, he says.

Get some feedback. After it's all said and done, it's okay to ask whether you're the right guy for the job. "When they say, 'Do you have any other questions?' at the end, say, 'One more: We've spent time together; how do you see my skill sets fitting with this job?' This works. Often they're very honest about your chances. It sure beats wondering," says Pachter.

Give thanks. Within the day, send a short thank-you note written in your most readable handwriting. If people often tell you they can't read your handwriting, have someone write it for you. Make sure your grammar and spelling are perfect.

"It has to be perfect. It's one of the ways that recruiters weed through the pile," says Pachter. "Done well, it's a very respectful way to reiterate your interest in the job, and how your skills fit."

Earning Your Boss's Respect

How to Be a Go-To Guy

Some might call it butt kissing. But those who take the time to study and learn their boss's intricacies—from body language and facial expressions to logic and concerns—are the men who eventually earn their boss's respect.

Just to be clear: We're *not* talking about butt kissing. Or brownnosing. Or boot licking. Or sucking up. This isn't about being a yes-man or mastering the art of empty flattery.

It's about making sure that you clearly understand what your boss wants and then doing your best to get the job done. From looking at criticism in a fresh, new way to meeting deadlines, here's a primer on the care and feeding of your boss.

Take the gift. If you're one of those people who immediately goes on the defensive when your boss makes a suggestion or even remotely criticizes one of your ideas, try to think of it as a gift. And we're not talking about those ill-fitting sweaters that your Aunt Mildred hands out every Christmas. "Defensive people cannot listen; therefore, defensive people cannot learn," says Darrel W. Ray, Ed.D., an organizational psychologist based in Kansas City, Kansas, and author of *Teaming Up.* "Look for the germ of truth. There is almost always some piece of truth in what somebody tells you. So rather than throwing away the baby with the bathwater, you need to listen and say, 'The boss is about to give me a gift. It may not be what I want, but at least he didn't tell five other people about this. He is

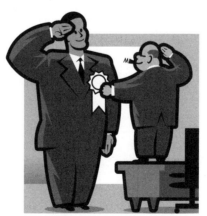

telling me personally; he is taking the courageous step of being honest with me.'"

Go to instant replay. Another way to short-circuit the defensiveness that can wreck your relationship is to repeat the feedback immediately after you get it. "The first words out of your mouth should be a repetition of what you heard, not your defense, not your argument," Dr. Ray says. "A lot of people resist that. They say, 'When I repeat it, I'm admitting to it.' Not at all. You're just repeating what you heard, and that is respectful. It gives you a chance to clarify something you may have misheard."

Try a different vantage point. For certain people, everything seems to come down to the same, simple question: "What's in it for me?" It sounds selfish, and it is. But if you turn it around, it can be an extremely useful way of getting things done. The idea is to focus on what you can do to benefit the other person. "Let's face it: Life is selling," says George Walther, a communications consultant based in Seattle and author of *Power Talking.* "Anytime that you're communicating with another person, you're selling your point of view...(but) what's important to me is not necessarily important to the other person. What's really important is what's important to *them.*"

Know when to hold them. You won't earn the respect of a healthy boss serving as the office doormat. But there are times when it pays to keep your mouth shut, says Sharon Anthony Bower, president of Confidence Training, based in Stanford, California, and co-author of *Asserting Yourself.* "If you're in a meeting and you're the new employee and your boss in some way slighted you, you should simply be quiet," Bower says. "But don't be quiet forever. It's important to go to your boss perhaps the next day—not a week from now, but pretty soon—and describe what happened from your point of view, express your feelings and your thoughts, specify a behavior change, and lay out the positive consequences for getting an agreement." (For more on proper assertiveness techniques, see Humility on page 56.)

Take a stand. There's a difference between sounding like a malcontent and providing honest feedback that's contrary to workplace opinion. The key is understanding that some bosses are more receptive to constructive criticism than others. If your boss wants your honest opinion, give it to him. Just be aware that if you're constantly disagreeing with him, you run the risk of being perceived as a malcontent—regardless of your good intentions. So pick your battles wisely, and present any criticism you have in private—not in front of others. "A good boss will respect that," says Alan Weiss, Ph.D., founder of Summit Consulting Group in East Greenwich, Rhode Island, and author of *Whatever Happened to Excellence?*

Work That Body

What you say to the boss is only part of the respect equation. It's how you say it that really makes a difference. Even if you're uttering all the right words, you could be undermining yourself by your body language. Here are some things to keep in mind.

Position yourself for success. Slouching is not a trait you link with respect. And with good reason. When sitting with the boss, you should keep your back straight, but lean slightly forward to show how interested you are by whatever he or she is saying. Standing? Also lean forward slightly. Maintain comfortable eye contact as he speaks, averting your gaze every 10 seconds or so, says Marjorie Brody, a certified speaking professional, co-author of the *Prentice Hall Complete Business Etiquette Handbook*, and president of Brody Communications, a business and

> ## No Tell, Noel?
>
> Your boss has been greeting guests at his office Christmas party with a piece of mistletoe mysteriously wedged in his teeth. Or his breath would kill a reindeer. Or his wife has a run in her stocking two feet long. What do you do?
>
> "Be direct and be discreet," says Mary Mitchell, author of *The Complete Idiot's Guide to Etiquette* as well as the "Ms. Demeanor" column syndicated to newspapers throughout the United States. "Get the person out of earshot of other people and say, 'You have something in your teeth' in the same tone of voice that you would use to say, 'It's raining outside.' "
>
> If you don't know the boss that well, find someone who does to break the news.

communications skills training company in Elkins Park, Pennsylvania.

Nix annoying habits. Hand wringing, finger tapping, pen clicking, or chair swiveling while the boss is talking makes you look like you either just busted out of Sing-Sing or you're not very confident. Neither command respect or a fat Christmas bonus, Brody says.

Reflect success. Mirroring works for cops trying to ease tension, and it can work for you when you're spending quality time with the boss, Brody advises. If he crosses his legs, do the same. If he loosens his tie, ditto. By affecting similar posture, you're saying, "I'm with you all the way, Chief."

Don't be a doorman. If he's talking on the phone when you arrive, don't poke your head in every 15 seconds or start wandering the halls. Some bosses pull this trick to unnerve you, Brody says. Catch his eye and shrug your shoulders once as if to say, "Now or later?" If he raises a finger, hover for a minute—max. If he shrugs back, head to your office and wait for him to call.

Keep him engaged. When the boss responds to your groundbreaking idea for battery-operated paper clips by taking off his glasses, rubbing his eyes, and leaning back in his chair, suffice it to say you haven't struck pay dirt. But don't give up yet. Re-engage your boss and his attention by placing written support material on the desk in front of him and saying something like, "I know this sounds unusual. Let me take you down the path for a moment," says Linda Blackman, president of The Executive Image, a Pittsburgh-based business communications company, and co-author of *The Sales Coach: Selling Tips from the Pros.*

Coming Through in the Clutch

Nothing warms a pesky boss's heart more than when one of his charges makes or beats a deadline. Experts aren't exactly sure why this is so, although some link it to the megalomania often associated with bossdom, while others believe it's such a rare occurrence that it almost takes on a mythical quality—like the Red Sox winning the World Series.

But forget the boss for a minute. (We know—if only it were that easy.) Who doesn't want to be known as a guy who performs well under pressure? At least in our fantasy lives, we all want to be Joe Montana or Michael Jordan, pulling out an improbable victory as the clock winds down. Mastering deadlines, then, offers a powerful one-two punch: You earn your boss's trust and respect, not to mention undying gratitude if the stakes are high enough, and you elevate your own self-esteem. Talk about a win-win proposition.

Here's how to become Mr. Clutch.

Say your goodbyes. Does your boss—or anyone else—have a habit of lingering about your office like a musty odor, telling war stories and burning up valuable man hours? You can respectfully clear the air, so to speak, by effectively spelling out the benefit of his absence. Walther offers this scenario: "Let's say your boss's name is Dave. 'Excuse me, Dave. I know that you're eager for me to complete my project on time, and I want to do that for you. I'm expecting to talk with one of the subcontractors about one minute from now. So what I would love to do is continue our conversation later so that I can get this done on time for you.' In other words, it's not, 'I have something I need to do,' but rather, 'In order for me to complete what you would like to get done, I am going to break now for that.' The back end is, 'I want to continue our conversation, let's do that after.'"

Beat the clock. The best way to beat the boss's clock is to simply set a date that you can easily meet or exceed. "Here's the secret: Always promise less than what you can do," Walther says. "Then when you get it done early, he's going to say, 'Gosh, he's always doing more than he said he was going to do.'" How does that look on paper? Suppose you know you can complete a project by 5:00 P.M. Thursday. Tell the boss you'll have it in by noon Friday. Work like a dog to get it done, and then put it on his desk after he leaves on Thursday. When he comes in the next morning, he has his finished project and you'll have his respect.

Advise ASAP. If you discover that you can't make your self-imposed deadline, you could wait until it's due and then switch into Full Excuse Mode—complete with commensurate levels of groveling and brownnosing. Or you could do some serious damage control by advising the boss as soon as you know there's a problem. "Once again, let's get into the other person's shoes," Walther says. "There is going to be a delay that's going to cause an inconvenience for your boss. What's in it for him? You would say something like, 'I had a commitment to get that proposal done by Thursday. I have two other estimates that could help save us some money—or whatever—but they are not available until Friday. So I would like to recommit. I will have that proposal to you no later than the end of the day Monday.'"

The Respect of Your Peers

Proving Yourself at Work

It was the novelist and critic Gore Vidal who once commented: "Whenever a friend succeeds, a little something in me dies." Admit it, you know the feeling. We all do. And perhaps nowhere is that more true than in the workplace.

As any newly minted vice-president will tell you, hard work and great ideas will help land you not only an executive parking spot but also the scornful looks of some jealous peers. It seems unfair that the very conduct that earns you the respect of your boss and a fast-track to promotion also can result in backbiting and jealousy among your co-workers. But then, nobody ever said life is fair.

Jealousy may be the main factor that can rob you of the respect of your co-workers, but it certainly isn't the only one. Constant complaining, talking about people behind their back, and contrasting personal styles also can breed disrespect. There are, however, actions you can take today to counter these common workplace maladies so that you are judged worthy of respect by the jury of your peers.

Promoting Harmony

All of your hard work finally paid off. You've been promoted. And suddenly, the guys you play hoops with at lunchtime each week treat you differently. What you sense isn't respect. It's more like...resentment. What's going on? After all, if one of them had

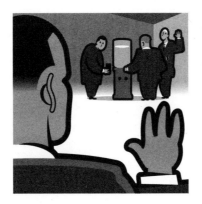

gotten the promotion, you'd be happy for them. Wouldn't you?

Even among friends, the success of one can fuel insecurity in another. "All jealous people basically feel they're not as good as others," says Paul Hauck, Ph.D., a psychologist in Rock Island, Illinois, and author of *Overcoming the Rating Game.*

Some of your peers see your achievement and feel like there must be something lacking in themselves. "They rate themselves by your success," Dr. Hauck says. " 'He got the promotion, I didn't. He is better than I am. I am insanely jealous of that other person. Why didn't it happen to me?' They believe that getting a promotion makes you a better person."

One of the ways you can show that you're worthy of your new title is by handling the situation with skill. Here are a few suggestions.

Lose the cape. As tempting as it may be to display your superhuman skills and ambitions to these lesser mortals, it's the last thing you want to do. "You need to exude the idea that you're no better than they," Dr. Hauck says. "Underplay your success if you can."

Encourage the envious. Say you have a buddy who's happy for you, but disappointed in his own apparent lack of success. He will respect you even more if you take the time to encourage him. Dr. Hauck suggests telling him, "I like the stuff you're doing. If it were up to me, you'd be next."

Corner the market on motivation. Behind almost every great fighter is a great cornerman, a trainer who prepares his boxer for success and keeps him motivated and focused during the bout. Even if you're now in the corner office, you can knock out office jealousy by making it clear to a disgruntled co-worker that you're in his corner. "Your attitude and actions should underscore the idea that you'd like to help move him ahead in his career as much as you can," says Dr. Hauck.

Corral Complaining

If you're the kind of guy who confuses honesty with bitching and moaning, break out your violin: People not only don't respect you but they don't like you, and they can see you coming a mile away. "These are the attributes that people associate with complainers: negativity, moodiness, dogmatism, and—surprise—pessimism," says Robin Kowalski, Ph.D., associate professor of psychology at Western Carolina University in Cullowhee, North Carolina. "And if you exhibit those kinds of characteristics, according to our research, you're going to be pretty well disliked."

So why do some guys complain? It turns out that the old *Saturday Night Live* sketch about an annoying family known as The Whiners was probably right on the money. Complaining is probably, in part, another charming parental legacy. "If your parents were chronic complainers, then in all likelihood you're going to have some of those traits," Dr. Kowalski says.

But you can break the habit. Here are three steps Dr. Kowalski recommends.

Find someone who cares. If you must complain, for Pete's sake, find someone who cares and isn't going to blab the sad tale all over creation. "I think the best advice is to be more discriminating," Dr. Kowalski says. "You don't want to alienate everyone you talk to. If you're discriminating, not only do you have to think about whom you're going to complain to but you also might even reconsider complaining entirely."

Get a real greeting. If your peers dart into their offices and cubicles as you walk past, it might be because you've failed to master Greeting 101. For example, if Walter from marketing says, "How are you?" he doesn't really want to hear about your ingrown toenails or the fact that the transmission fell out of your minivan on your way to Disney World. In fact,

there's a good chance that the only reason Walter asked you how you are was to give *himself* an opportunity to brag about his trip to Barbados with his new girlfriend, who—by the way—was just named Ms. September. Now that you know the game, simply answer "Great" and keep moving. If you're greeting others, "Good to see you" is a lot less nosy than "How are you?" and gives people a warm fuzzy—plus, *you'll* get fewer sob stories.

Get a clue. Suppose you unload your misery on the guy in the next dump truck—a tale of woe so dreadful that even this tattoo-wearing, beer-drinking behemoth is speechless. When the big guy finally weighs in with his opinion, it's a good idea just to listen carefully and then shut up. "A woman will stand there and keep listening, but the man will give you a problem-solving response and expect you to deal with it," Dr. Kowalski says. "If you keep complaining, it's like...'I already told you what to do, man. Move on.'"

Making It Work

There are other things you can do to enhance the respect of your peers. There also are things you can *not* do that will boost your standing. It's important to know the difference. Here are four suggestions from our experts.

Keep your ears open. You don't have to become the office psychologist or spend countless hours listening to sob stories. But guys who are willing to listen to their peers are so rare, you'll earn respect practically by default.

"Most people are poor listeners," says organizational psychologist Dr. Darrel W. Ray. "There is a tremendous amount of miscommunication that takes place in American business. People just don't want to listen to each other. And that leads to rudeness and disrespect...the whole social system breaks down."

Abolish "aboutism." What's worse than pretending someone doesn't exist? How about talking about them behind their back, a practice Dr. Ray calls aboutism.

"It's rampant in most workplaces. We all do it in the lunchroom and the break room, and we do it after work...during meetings and after meetings," Dr. Ray says. "Talking about people, complaining about them, rather than going to that person. In order to gain respect, you cannot engage in that kind of behavior. It destroys respect of any kind."

Be a behavioral scientist. You—and your stomach—would probably be pretty upset if your co-worker showed up an hour late to relieve you for your dinner break. But you'll have a better chance of helping him change if you can focus on his behavior rather than on him. "If I say, 'You didn't get back until 8:10 P.M.,' that is behavioral. You can observe that. But if I say, 'Bob, you're always late coming back from break,' that is not behavioral. Focus on what the behavior was and not the person. It's not the person that's bad. It's the behavior that hurts the company or hurts the team," says Dr. Ray.

Respect the other guy's style. Put two extremely talented, yet very different, people together and two things can happen. They can complement and challenge each other, producing work that exceeds what either could do individually (see Lennon and McCartney), or they could wind up at each other's throats, unable to stand even being in the same room together (see Lennon and McCartney). The key is to respect each other's differences and styles.

"You have to be somewhat understanding of the other's quirks and habits, moods, their best times to work, things like that," says Robert R. Butterworth, Ph.D., a trauma consultant and president of Contemporary Psychology Associates in Los Angeles.

Belittlers, Be Gone

One common way we let respect slip away is by using phrases that communications consultant George Walther calls belittlers.

"The idea of power talking isn't that you boost yourself and make yourself better than you are but, rather, that you give yourself appropriate credit," Walther says. "And you can't do that when you are belittling yourself." Two of the most common belittlers are:

"I'm just..." You can really bring yourself down a few notches in the eyes of your peers by frequently saying, "I'm just (fill in the blank)." "There is no reason to ever say, 'I am just anything,' " Walther advises. "It's quite common for a secretary taking a message to say, 'Well, gee, I don't know his availability. I'm just his assistant.' Compare that to 'I'm his assistant. I will be glad to check his availability and get back to you.' There's no question which sounds better."

"You'll have to excuse..." You can really raise questions about your competency by using this phrase. It does not one but two detrimental things: It draws attention to the things that you didn't want the other person to notice *and*, at no extra charge, makes it look like you feel guilty. "They may not have thought, 'My gosh, what a mess this is!' but they will when you say, 'Oh, you'll have to excuse the condition of my office.' I say fix it or forget about it. If you don't like the way your office looks, either clean it up or stop apologizing to others and just get on with your life. Odds are that they aren't going to notice anyway," Walther says.

If side-by-side collaboration is too intense, maybe that's why God invented fax machines and modems.

You're the Boss

Gaining Respect from Employees

You have the title, the corner office, and a paycheck that screams Platinum American Express—the credit card without that pesky preset spending limit. What more could you ask for?

Well, if you're the boss and you treat your employees with contempt, how about infamy? Consider this entry in a national Best Boss/Worst Boss contest that spawned the book (what else?) *Best Boss, Worst Boss.*

"After saying his good nights to the office (around 3:00 P.M.),...he would then return by sneaking up the back stairway. Ever so quietly, he would unlock the supply-closet door, go inside, and close the door. For the next 2 hours he would stand inside the closet with the door closed and the light off, listening to what employees said..."

It's probably safe to say that even when the lights *are* on, there's nobody home in this boss's office. But sad to say, he's not the only one. In this same contest, the submissions describing boneheaded bosses not only outnumber the ones describing good guys but they also detail some even more horrifying incidents, including:

- "Despite being a millionaire, my boss...often asked another supervisor to pop boils on his large, sweaty body."
- "Our boss makes employees stand in front of his office window with hand raised, indicating that they need to use the bathroom."
- "She loves to fire people on Christmas Eve.... In fact, she draws childish pictures of the people she fires, tapes the

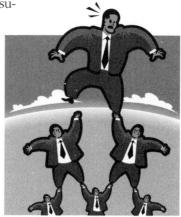

pictures to their empty chairs, and makes fun of the 'departed' employees."

Boss Tips

Surely it doesn't come as a surprise that some bosses feel it's necessary to exert control through deceit, humiliation, and degradation. But are more subtle forms of disrespect any less disrespectful? Probably not, says Jim Miller, author of *Best Boss, Worst Boss* and *The Corporate Coach.* "No matter what you do, if you don't have happy employees who feel like they're respected, they aren't going to treat your customers right. And then you're out of business," he says.

Nor is it enough to attend leadership or motivational courses, although they definitely have their place. "These are fun and interesting, but they don't get to the heart of the matter," says therapist Dr. Brian DesRoches, author of *Your Boss Is Not Your Mother.* "You have to dig deeper to make sure that your entire manner conveys respect."

Here are some simple, yet powerful, ways to make that happen.

Ditch the desk. There are a few days when it might be okay to hide behind a giant wooden desk—like, say, if you forget to wear your slacks to work. But a balanced, respectful boss doesn't need to assert his authority with office furniture. He comes out and around that shrine to his position and sits beside his employees when they visit. Not only that but also he'll listen to what they have to say and take action if he can—even though just listening is often enough, says Stephen J. Holoviak, former director of the Frehn Center for Management at Shippensburg University.

Toss the regal trappings. Okay, maybe some of us would be willing to kiss the Pope's ring or bow for the Queen of England. But bosses who expect us to bow and scrape at the company picnic, Christmas party—heck, even in the hallway—generate fear and loathing, not respect. "When you walk down the hall, your employees shouldn't tense up and stop what they're doing. You should greet them by name with a smile and apologize to them if you're interrupting," says Holoviak.

Loosen your grip. What are you, a boss or an extra in the movie *Backdraft*? If you want to fight office fires, volunteer for the local rescue squad. If you want your employees to grow and develop, empower them to handle tough situations, even during a crisis, and they'll give you better-quality work. As a bonus, you'll also earn their respect, says Holoviak. "The more successful they are, the more successful you are."

Prune your personnel handbook. A telling comparison of a department of corrections guide for prisoners and several company personnel handbooks revealed that each had about the same number of items. If the "don'ts" come close to outnumbering the "do's" in your shop, you have a problem that only a change of corporate attitude can cure, says Holoviak.

Assume the position. The big Kahuna not only has the biggest board on the beach but also the willingness to hang tough when the surf gets rough. "You might have to shoulder blame sometimes," says Dr. DesRoches. "This could hurt you with the company, no question about it. But it's going to make your employees more loyal to you. They'll follow you anywhere."

Share your vision. If George Bush's failure to understand or articulate "the vision thing" cost him the White House, what makes you think that you're going to hang on to power? "If you want people to buy in to your ideas, you have to give them your vision for the

Best Bosses

"There are some really fine bosses out there. Unfortunately, all you seem to hear about are the jerks," says Jim Miller, author of *Best Boss, Worst Boss* and *The Corporate Coach*. So here are some examples of what the good guys are doing. What strikes us about these testimonials, submitted by the thousands for an annual Best Boss/Worst Boss contest, is that a little kindness really seems to make a big impression.

- "If we stay late or make a suggestion he likes, he is quick to praise and thank us. I've never heard him raise his voice or degrade a person.... The warehouse staff is treated to surprise lunches, doughnuts for breakfast, even free tickets to local events."

- "Many times he would call my wife for permission to keep me at the office for some overtime work. He would always remember to send her a thank-you for her sacrifice and contribution to my career."

- "Instead of using impersonal formalities such as 'staff,' his memos are addressed to 'teammates' or 'friends.' "

- "One summer day, he announced that he had arranged for someone to answer the phone, and he was taking us to the movies! He even bought the popcorn."

organization and their role in it," Holoviak says. "What unique skills do they have to contribute and how do you intend to help maximize those contributions?"

Share your success. Bonuses, trips to exotic locales, stock options—these are the kinds of perks that make employees weep with joy. But even if your company can't afford such extravagances, you can still catch people doing good things and reward them. Ice cream parties, a movie ticket or two, even a certificate that simply says they did a fine job, all work wonders, Miller says.

Public Speaking

Talking about Respect

In Public Speaking 101, you learned the essentials of communicating effectively to a group: Keep your energy level high, speak clearly, and perhaps most important, at all times make absolutely certain that your fly is zipped up.

Now you may think that there's a better way to gain respect from an audience than simply appearing to be a reasonably normal human being. But acting like a regular guy during a presentation may actually be one of the quickest routes, says Dianna Booher, author of *Communicate with Confidence.*

"The best way to win over an audience right away is to show them a vulnerability. Let them see that you are genuine," Booher says. "Typically, you want to find something that you have in common with them or use some kind of self-effacing humor. Those are two good ways."

A Smooth Talker

You want the audience to be hanging on your every word—as long as you're not the one left hanging when all is said and done. Cheer up. Giving an effective speech or presentation is a surefire way to earn respect in the workplace. Here's how you can master the art of public speaking.

Start with the good stuff. The once-upon-a-time approach to communication works great for fairy tales (such as bedtime stories, George Lucas films, and most political convention speeches). But when it comes to making your talk count, consider hitting your audience with your punch line first.

Most speakers make the mistake of taking their audience through the whole history of the topic before concluding with what it is that they want the audience to do. It's much more effective to lay it on the line at the outset, Booher says. "In the inverted form of presentation, you tell them, 'This is what I want you to approve, buy, consider, contribute, or whatever.' You give them the bottom-line message up front—what action you want from the audience—and then go back and persuade them to do it," she says.

Ask the right questions. Sweaty palms. Heart palpitations. Spots in front of your eyes. Delusions of grandeur. Your first date with Vendela? No, just another corporate presentation about to start in a boardroom somewhere in America. The reason: Lots of guys are focusing on themselves before the speech and not their audience, Booher says.

"They're thinking, 'What if I'm embarrassed? What if I blow it? What if they ask me a question that I don't know the answer to?' " she says. If this sounds like you-know-who, remind yourself that they asked you to do this because you have some information these people need to know. But if you really want to give yourself the third degree, try these questions instead: What does my audience need to know? How can I help them use it? How will their lives be better after they have this information?

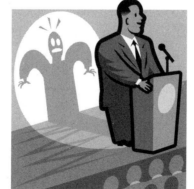

"Asking these kinds of questions will help you get rid of the self-consciousness that detracts from your presentation," Booher says. As an added bonus, focusing on your audience's needs will force you to prepare an even more impressive presentation.

Move around. Nervous speakers tend to resort to one of two extremes. There's what is called the nervous speaker's dance, in which you hop from foot to foot like you haven't visited a urinal since the Eisenhower administration. Then there's the death grip—locking onto the lectern, unable to budge until someone pries your cold, gnarled fingers loose.

Obviously, neither commands respect. The most effective technique for releasing pent-up energy is to move naturally around the room. "When you tense up, you shake more and it becomes more apparent. So to get rid of that, you should just move," Booher advises. "Don't pace, but stroll—up one side of the room while you make a point. Then go back to make another. Pick up a flip chart marker if you're going to mark something. Just moving around the room allows the tension to ooze out, if you will, and takes the quiver out of your voice."

Be body-wise. Keep your hands out of your pockets, where they might be tempted to rattle keys or coins. And you don't want to cross your arms or put your hands on your hips unless you're emphasizing a point. "Being more aware of where your feet are and what you're doing with your arms and hands is key," says Marjorie Brody, a certified speaking professional and president of Brody Communications, a business and communications skills training company.

Forget faking it. When the clock runs out on your preparation time, the temptation sometimes is to loft the linguistical equivalent of a Hail Mary pass and hope for the best. You know the drill: trying to finesse them with some jargon or tossing out some time-honored generalities. But there's probably no quicker way to lose the respect of an audience. "They smell blood when somebody asks you a question and you can't answer it. Then they tend to discount everything else that you said," Booher warns. There is a bold alternative: telling the truth. "Say, 'You know, I don't really know the answer to that; I probably should have gotten those figures together before I came, but I didn't. Let me check and get back to you'—instead of trying to bluff your way through. Once you have lost that credibility, you can almost never regain it."

Act the underdog. If the questions get really nasty, there's no need to retaliate. In fact,

you're better off playing the underdog, Booher says. If you think that you'll lose the audience's respect unless you fire back a smart-aleck response, think again. "Actually, just the opposite is true," she says. Americans have a profound respect for the underdog. We root for the underdog. So nothing increases your stature as much as remaining calm and collected and composed when answering a question that was put to you in a hostile, put-down manner."

One of the best ways to respond is to quickly lower and reduce the inflection in your voice, eliminate your hand gestures, and step away from the obnoxious party. "We're not talking about giving in to them. It just means that you state your opposite opinion or your answer or response in a nonintimidating way. And that becomes a startling contrast to the attack that has been made," Booher says.

Recover quickly. Let's assume the worst. You just went off on the guy who has been giving you a hard time. Despite what you may think, all is not lost. "Just back up and laugh at yourself," says Booher. "Try something like, 'I guess you can tell I feel strongly about that point,' and laugh. Then come back with an even tone. But I think you need to call attention to it because if someone else calls attention to it, *that's* when it becomes a problem."

Make the material yours. There's no telling how long it may take to prepare for your presentation. A seasoned pro like Booher still studies for 2 hours to make sure a special 1½-hour speech for Wall Street execs sounds polished and professional—even though she has done it before. But whatever you do, don't memorize the material word-for-word.

"I am not advocating going in there by the seat of your pants," says Booher. "Your opening sentence and your transition from point to point can be memorized and polished. Your opening minute or two should be polished and memorized. And your last minute or two should be polished. But the elaboration on each point should be close to extemporaneous. That always should be fresh. You never want to memorize. It sounds memorized."

Respect for a Salesman

Turning Your Cursed Job into a Respectable Profession

"Salesman" is an eight-letter dirty word.

It brings to mind the image of a greasy-haired guy with a fake smile and bad cologne who talks too fast and bullies and lies to get you to buy something you don't need or want. Not exactly the kind of stuff respect is made out of.

So, for a salesman to earn respect, he can't let on that he's trying to sell something. Got that? Don't look like, act like, or sound like a salesman. "If you do what most salespeople do, you'll be as successful as most salespeople are, which is not all that successful," says Craig Arnoff, president of The Sales Alliance, a sales development firm that has improved the sales revenues of more than 150 firms throughout the United States.

Playing with the Pros

What do typical salespeople do? They peddle. They call or visit as many people as they can, talk as fast as they can about their product, and pray that someone, anyone will say the magic words: "How much?" About 80 percent of the time, they get a door slammed in their face or a phone slammed into their ear, says Arnoff.

"Most of us as consumers really never get to see true sales professionals. Instead, we see the most poorly trained segment of sales society," says Michael O'Horo, the son of a salesman, who has worked in sales for 25 years and developed *The Practice Builder*, a program based in

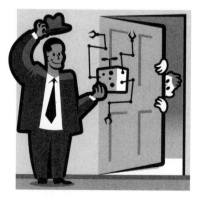

Washington, D.C., that is used to help lawyers better sell their services.

It's really not difficult to change from disrespected peddler to a successful sales professional. Here's how to earn respect and make more sales.

Look the part. If you are going to sell to construction workers, don't wear a suit. If you are selling to lawyers, don't wear jeans. You want to dress and talk as similarly as your customer as possible, says Joachim de Posada, Ph.D., an international industrial psychologist who teaches seminars on sales, management, leadership, and team building and author of numerous videotapes, including *Psychology Applied to Sales*. Otherwise, you'll be viewed as a conniving outsider.

Find an opening. The first few seconds of a sale can be the most crucial, especially over the phone when it's too easy for someone to hang up. To quickly show the person you have something valuable to say, the first words out of your mouth should outline why you are calling. Then, immediately tell the customer why he should listen. And finally, ask permission to continue, says Dr. de Posada.

Ingratiate yourself. One of the best things you can do to quickly win someone's respect as well as break the ice? Compliment him, says Dr. de Posada. If you are standing in his entryway, marvel at how well his hardwood floors look or compliment him on his lawn. At the office, start up a conversation about his trophies or prestigious educational certificates.

Anthony R. Pratkanis, Ph.D., professor of psychology at the University of California at Santa Cruz and author of *The Age of Propaganda: The Everyday Use and Abuse of Persuasion*, actually has studied how well sucking up can work. He and other researchers walked up to random people on the street, complimented them on their attire, and then hit them up with a request to donate to charity. "Not only would they contribute to the charity but they also were willing to help out someone else with a request just a short time later. Ingratiation puts people in a good mood," says Dr. Pratkanis.

Avoid premature presentation. When you immediately launch into a product pitch, it makes the customer feel like you have a huge need to sell this product, thus something must be wrong with it. Plus, as soon as you pitch what you are trying to sell, the guy decides if he wants to buy or not and the whole conversation is over. "Your presentation will always be the last thing you do because once you give it, the customer makes a decision," says O'Horo. "The sooner you present, the sooner you are out."

Probe. Shut up and let the customer talk, says Dr. de Posada. Use questions to guide the customer to your product. For instance, start by asking open-ended questions to get the person talking. Then, when the guy mentions anything remotely related to what you are selling, direct him to your chosen topic with closed questions—where the person can answer yes or no or choose among options.

The technique helps you sell because the open-ended questions will reveal what that guy is already willing to buy. He may tell you that he's worried about his kid getting into college. If you're selling encyclopedias, tutoring, or some other education product, you're in luck. And it earns you respect because all you've done is helped the guy out.

Listen. It will make the person feel like you care. You can prove you are listening by summarizing what someone just said, says Arnoff.

Match your words to your actions. A famous study during the 1970s found that people pay attention to 7 percent of our words, 38 percent of our volume, and 55 percent of our body movements. So if you are telling

Shaking Up Respect

In putting this chapter together, we uncovered tons of proven ways to make a sale. We also found some methods that were a bit, shall we say, underhanded.

Like the handshake. This universal symbol of trust can be used to hook customers into buying something they may not want, says the University of California's Dr. Anthony R. Pratkanis, author of *The Age of Propaganda: The Everyday Use and Abuse of Persuasion*. Most people honor their commitments. So if you make someone feel like they have made a commitment to buy your product—even if he really hasn't—he probably won't let you down, says Dr. Pratkanis. For instance, getting someone to fill out paperwork that requires a signature or prematurely forcing your hand into his for a "let's shake on it" will make him feel obligated to buy, even if he doesn't want to.

If you're the kind of guy who rarely confronts the same customer twice, you can probably get away with this stuff and not worry about damaging your respect—as long as you can live with yourself. Just remember, we're not advocating that you go out and do this stuff. We're just letting you know it works.

someone that "this is the most exciting thing since Tickle Me Elmo," but you say it without the slightest smile or eye twinkle, you'll look like a big fat liar. You want to make sure to smile, keep eye contact, and provide a firm handshake, says Dr. de Posada.

Stick around when the going gets tough. Once you sell something, be sure to make amends if something goes wrong, says Dr. Pratkanis. If a zipper breaks, send a replacement product or get the original fixed. Providing such help not only mollifies someone's anger but it also makes a person feel that you are someone who can be depended on in the future.

At a Business Meeting

Your Showcase to Shine

It has been several years now since Alan Caruba, the fun-loving founder of The Boring Institute in Maplewood, New Jersey, compiled his organization's official list of the 10 most mind-numbing activities. To no one's surprise, holding steady at number four (just behind standing in line, doing laundry, and commuting): meetings.

"Easily half to three-quarters of all meetings are so unstructured and poorly planned that they're an utter and total waste of time and productivity," Caruba says.

If meetings themselves have a deservedly bad rap, there's little hope for the man responsible for wasting other people's time. "A guy who holds a lot of meetings that have no agenda, no structure, and who fails to achieve a consensus will quickly become an object of company-wide ridicule," Caruba says.

Meeting the Challenge

As long as you're not the honcho running the show, a meandering meeting could open the door to opportunity for you. In fact, with a few carefully executed maneuvers, your corporate stock could soar.

Just be careful, says Lyle Sussman, Ph.D., professor of management at the University of Louisville and co-author of *Smart Moves for People in Charge.* "You never execute a smart move unless you feel like you can pull it off," he says.

We won't bore you by bringing up the obvious stuff,

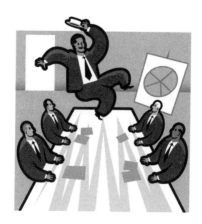

like urging you to get there on time and to never drool on the person seated next to you. But the rest of these tips could very well make your next meeting something to look forward to.

Be prepared. In today's overworked office environment, it's all that most meeting participants can do to trudge in and take their seats without collapsing into a coma. Instead of remaining in the ranks of the undead, why not actually spend a few minutes preparing for the next powwow? "The more homework you do, the more background research you have, the better prepared you will be—and that is going to stand out," Dr. Sussman says.

Take it to the next level. If you really want to be ahead of the game, you might even consider huddling with some of your fellow workers before the meeting. "One way to do it would be bouncing ideas off of trusted colleagues and mentors, but it's also valuable to talk to other participants prior to the meeting to get some sense of where they fall on issues," says Dr. Sussman. For an even greater advantage, consider developing hypothetical scenarios and role-playing them. "Imagining how the meeting will progress if this is said or that is said is light-years ahead of what most people do. And it would also help you determine when to interject your comments," he says.

Seat yourself. There was a scene in the movie *Disclosure* in which Michael Douglas's character was forced to sit through a meeting of high-powered execs in a chair that was about six sizes too small for the conference table. The result: He looked like a weenie. Forget the fact that Douglas's vindictive boss (played by Demi Moore) purposely changed the meeting time to help tank his career. The point here is that you want to land the best seat in the house— and that happens to be directly across from the meeting leader.

"That's where you can have the most impact," says Dr. Sussman. "You'll be able to read the leader's eye contact and nonverbal cues. And the more nonverbal cues that you can pick up from the person leading the meeting, the better." There's another even more subtle benefit beyond seeing what he's doing: *He's* going to be looking at you—and as a result, he may even provide a forum for your views. "If you're looking at him intently, maintaining eye contact, if that leader has any sensitivity at all, he'll notice that you are ready to speak and then introduce your comment in a very subtle, nonmanipulative way," he says.

Weigh in with impact. We all know people who speechify at meetings with the gusto of a 12th-term congressman, somehow hoping to sway you with their self-serving views. Or at least talk you to death. *They* might be confused about how to command respect at a meeting, but you don't have to be.

"You want to say something that actually makes a difference to the final outcome rather than just saying something simply to be heard," Dr. Sussman says. To best pick your shot, only say something that gets the meeting back on track or brings the question at hand into focus. Then shut up. "The irony is that the person who talks the most isn't necessarily the most influential. It's the person who says what should be heard," says Dr. Sussman.

Time your talk. For maximum impact, save your comments until near the end of the meeting. "I think the last comments are the ones that get remembered," Dr. Sussman says. "Just when you think the group is most frustrated, just when you think they're looking for the insightful comment, just when you think they are waiting for the idea that will never come, that's when you ought to trot it out."

Take a stand. If you want to make a bold statement that you're a player to be reckoned with, consider standing when making your point—even if everyone else is sitting. "I have seen it and coached it and, at times, recommend it," Dr. Sussman says. "There are some who just think better when they're on their feet." But rather than pacing the floor like an NBA coach with a team in serious foul

trouble, consider opting for a chalk talk. "If there's a flip chart in the room and no one has used it, that might be a perfect opportunity to get up and use it—even if you're just using it as an excuse to get you on your feet. I would give this one a great deal of thought before I tried it, but it can work. It can make you look assertive," says Dr. Sussman.

Dare to summarize. If the meeting leader allows discussion to meander all over the place, summarizing the comments of the last few speakers—and then introducing what you believe is the common thread tying them together—can be extremely effective, says Dr. Sussman. "It's not just your point; it's your point in the context of three to four preceding comments," he says. Such a presentation makes it sound like you have the focus and clarity of a laser beam and the analytical skills of Mr. Spock.

Ask for an executive summary. When an already-long monologue turns into an outright filibuster, some will nap. Others will dream of leaving the room. But you can tactfully and respectfully help wrap up the discussion by asking for what's called an executive summary, says Dr. Sussman. "There are lots of people who ramble on and don't believe they are," he says. To help focus the discussion without embarrassing them, Dr. Sussman suggests interjecting something like, "Your comments are very helpful. In essence, what is your position?" Or, "If you were going to give an executive summary in about a minute, what would it be?"

Be a facilitator. Helping draw other people out during a meeting can not only win you kudos from your boss but it can also enhance your standing with your peers. "You can ask nonthreatening questions that tap their feelings like, 'Jack, what do you think about what Sam just said?' Or have them relate specific information in their field that they have at their fingertips or know off the top of their head. Something like, 'Tom, I know you just did that survey last week. Could you please summarize it briefly for the group?'" Dr. Sussman suggests. "You're trying to throw a high fast ball so they look good. And that will break the ice."

Handling Conflicts

Can't We All Just Get Along?

While "lean and mean" has become synonymous with the efficient, aggressive corporation, lots of employees and managers will tell you that it also describes an increasingly hostile and demanding workplace. Namely, *theirs*.

"The fact is that the American manager and employees have taken a shot over the past decade," says Dr. Alan Weiss of Summit Consulting Group and author of *Whatever Happened to Excellence?* "If I let go of 100 execs and middle managers...and I hire 400 hamburger flippers, you might call that a net gain of 300 jobs. I would call that a travesty."

Few hurt more than those who lose their jobs without just cause during such housecleanings. And those who remain? Although they may at first be grateful that they've been spared, they soon discover there's a high price for keeping their jobs. In this era of mergers and acquisitions, "camaraderie and pitching-in are going by the wayside because no one has any hint whether they're going to be axed anymore," says Dr. Robert R. Butterworth, a trauma consultant and president of Contemporary Psychology Associates. "Back-stabbing goes up. And so in a sense, it becomes a situation where no one is secure. And when you're not secure, that creates all sorts of problems, including anxiety."

Net result: We lose respect for the organization because we've lost its loyalty. Gross result: Conflict. And lots of it. From office shootings to corporate coups d'état, the headlines are filled with the aftermath—to say

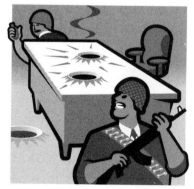

nothing of the soaring stress levels and frayed emotions of those who somehow cling to their jobs and sanity.

The Great Communicator

It only makes sense, then, that respect in the workplace is more important than ever. And when used to temper either our words or actions, respect not only helps diffuse the most volatile situations but also can prevent them.

"There's a new competitiveness in the workplace that doesn't just encourage emotional competence; it demands it," says Daniel Goleman, Ph.D., a behavioral sciences writer for the *New York Times* and author of *Emotional Intelligence.* "When emotionally upset, people cannot remember, learn, or make decisions clearly. This certainly can destroy careers, if not corporations."

While keeping our anger in check is key in handling conflict—and is another way of showing our respect for others—building respect into all our communications can benefit everyone.

"The basic issue here is: Are you just putting your communication out there, or are you responsible for making sure that it arrives in an understandable, respectful fashion?" says communications consultant George Walther. "The greater the responsibility that you take for the communications in your life, the bigger the payoff. An excellent communicator will take that responsibility."

In fact, small changes in speech can be one of the best ways to avoid conflict and show people that you respect their words and ideas. Here are some of the most common errors and how to fix them, according to Walther.

Consider more, disagree less. You simply may not agree with what the other guy is saying, but don't use the word *disagree* if you can avoid it. "People don't hear 'disagree.' They hear, 'He said: I'm wrong. My idea wasn't good...I used some faulty reasoning to reach my conclusion.' Now their energy goes not into hearing you, but into defending their position," Walther says. Instead, try: "I'd also like you to consider..." Using this simple phrase allows the other person to buy in and make their own contributions—without making them feel like a bonehead. "It's not 'my idea' or 'your idea.' It's 'Here's another idea,'" he says. "Let's look at both and we may come out with something that's even better."

Banish "misunderstanding." In the marketplace of ideas, there's little room for misunderstanding—the word, that is. Especially when *you're* responsible for making your message clear. "When you say, 'You don't understand,' again some magic transformation happens," says Walther. "The other person hears, 'You're stupid. Can't you figure this out? You have inferior intellect.' So never say, 'No, you are misunderstanding me.' It's much more effective to say, 'I didn't make that clear enough.'"

Avoid accusations. Really want to pick a fight? Accuse somebody of something. Interested in solving a problem without starting another? Say you're disappointed. "Saying, 'When you come in late, your tardiness does this to me...' sounds like an accusation. But if I switch it around and say, 'I feel disappointed. I feel frustrated by your tardiness,' then you can't argue with that. That's how I feel," Walther says.

"But" out. "Make a conscious decision to replace the word *but* with *and* as you talk with yourself and to others," Walther says. Where *but* focuses like a laser beam on differences, *and* allows ideas to peacefully co-exist—and hence, avoid conflict. Instead of saying, "You did a good job, but there's a small problem I need to talk with you about," try this:

To Boldly Go...

One of the Klingons on your Starship Enterprise has just attacked, and your physiological systems have raised the heat shields. But Scotty is in the engine room screaming that there's no more power—in this case, that you must keep your cool. For such situations, therapist Dr. Brian DesRoches, author of *Your Boss Is Not Your Mother*, recommends developing a rote response. Call it—if you're willing to endure our *Star Trek* analogy for one more second—your photon torpedo of respect.

"You want to honor your desire to get calm and at the same time acknowledge that the other person is very upset. What usually happens is that we take the bait, and in taking the bait, that person never changes and neither do we," Dr. DesRoches says. One possible stock answer: "I want to be able to give you a thoughtful answer to what is going on, and in order to do that, I have to think for myself and get back to you." Then leave the situation.

"You did a good job, and there's a small problem I need to talk with you about."

After the Battle Lines Have Been Drawn

When conflict erupts, some guys prepare to duke it out—verbally as well as physically. But unless you're auditioning for a Jackie Chan flick or The McLaughlin Group, that may not be the best approach. Here are some more respectful ways to handle conflict.

Explore, don't ignore. You wouldn't ignore a sucking chest wound, so why try to ignore conflict—which could very well lead to one? "Let's say you are talking to a customer who is disappointed about his experience with your product," Walther says. "You're going to hear inflamed language. You would rather be getting off the phone. Wrong. Terminating the conversation or shifting attention away doesn't end it. You're just capping it."

While the other person is still hot, ask them to tell you about the problem. "They have some feelings they need to get out," says Walther. "You're not going to be able to make headway with this person until they tell you more."

Let it blow. Telling someone to simmer down is likely to blow up in your face. "Doing that doesn't make the other person settle down...it just stifles them temporarily and that makes the explosion bigger later," Walther warns.

Hop the fence. The next step when dealing with the disgruntled: Build rapport by saying, "You know, we really want the same thing," Walther advises. "Hostile parties often visualize the two of you on opposite sides of a fence. You are the enemy. This is a showdown.... But if you say, 'Gosh, we really want the same thing,' they're going to see you in a new way."

Hand them the keys. We score major conflict resolution points when we let the other guy decide how to make the situation right. "Now here is the surprise: Most people are reluctant to do that when they are on the receiving end of a conflict because they think the other person will come up with some kind of outlandish, impossible claim," Walther says. The reality: Most people are more reasonable than that. In fact, they're probably going to ask for less than you are prepared to offer. "They just want to be heard, respected, and paid attention to," he says.

Learning the Other Language

Body language plays such an important role in creating and resolving conflict that law enforcement personnel are taught how to use it to help gain control in tense situations, says organizational psychologist Dr. Darrel W. Ray. But you can use the same skills whether you're getting a tongue-lashing from a subcontractor or mixing it up during the company softball game.

Play musical chairs. If you're seated and going face-to-face, one of the smartest things you can do is pick your chair up and move it around to the other person's side of the table. "Subliminally, the message is that you and I together, side-by-side, are going to use our mutual strengths against that problem out there," Walther says.

Be well-armed. We all know that folded arms can sometimes show a level of anger or distrust. The next time a conflict erupts, try to keep your arms at your sides. And when gesturing, do it slowly and gently with your palms open and up. "Pushing down with your hand or pushing away with your hand is a closing-off gesture. If I keep the palms of my hands up and open to you, that's a nondefensive gesture," Dr. Ray says.

Turn down the volume. The tendency during a disagreement is to raise your voice, yell, or, for some of us, foam at the mouth. Slobber if you must, but turning up your volume is a poor choice if you want to resolve conflict respectfully. "Fire can only get fueled if you fuel it," says Dr. Ray. On the other hand, "it's hard for someone to yell and scream and jump up and down if nobody is going to do that with them."

Meet your match. Ever notice that when you're enjoying yourself with a friend, you match each other's gestures or walk with your strides in sync? That demonstrates mirroring—another technique cops and other law enforcement types use during conflicts.

"If you're in an uproar, emotionally upset, then I'm going to mirror that on a lower level," Dr. Ray says. "If you're flailing about with your hands, then I might use my hands a little broader, but then use them less and less to create a less animated pace for you. I'll slow myself down...and I will reduce my gestures and lead you into a more rational conversation," says Dr. Ray.

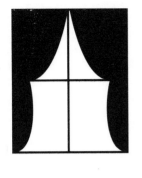

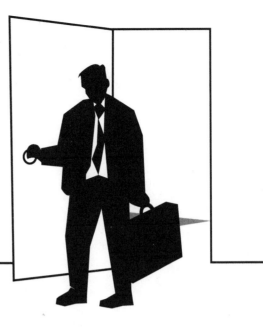

Part Four

Respect When You
Get Home

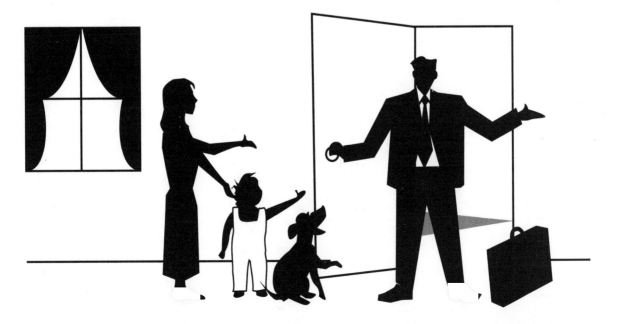

The Virtuous Son

Earning Respect from Your Parents

The defining moment in a man's life is not when he throws the winning touchdown pass. Or discovers the cure to a previously incurable disease. Or first locks eyes across a crowded room with the woman he knows he will marry (if only she'd lose that dimwit by her side with the family crest on his blazer). No, that one-in-a-gazillion moment of truth happens approximately nine months before he is even born, when his father's squiggling little sperm burrows its way into a tiny egg inside his mother. And through the miracle of creation, his life takes form.

This is our roundabout way of illustrating what psychologists tell us again and again: We are the sum of our parents. We are a blend of their genes. We pick up their vocabulary. Our values are their values, our gait theirs. Besides being our genetic benefactors, they are also our role models, our teachers. If they are often our heroes, they also are sometimes our anti-heroes.

What does all this have to do with earning their respect? Plenty, says Frank Pittman III, M.D., a psychiatrist and family therapist in Atlanta and author of *Man Enough: Fathers, Sons, and the Search for Masculinity.* "You begin to earn respect from your parents by first respecting how influential they have been in molding your personality," he says. "Then you live a life that they would respect—regardless of whether it's the life they would choose to live."

All in the Family

Earning your parents' respect is tricky business for both

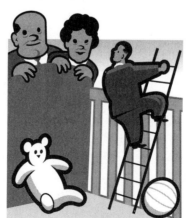

men and women. But for men it's even more complex.

With our mothers, it seems we earn their respect just by showing up. "In many a mother's eyes, no one will be as wonderful as her son," says Ann F. Caron, Ed.D., developmental psychologist and author of *Strong Mothers, Strong Sons: Raising the Next Generation of Men.* When a son senses that that "no one" includes his father, the family plot thickens. Does the term "Oedipus complex" ring any bells? That's the subconscious tangle psychoanalyst Sigmund Freud describes when a very young boy begins to see his mother as the object of his bubbling sexual urges and his father as his rival.

Most of us would call this hogwash, but "all sons at some point or another have sensed that they can get what they want from their mothers but not from their fathers," notes Dr. Pittman.

It is even more complex with our fathers. "Yearning to earn a father's respect is one of the most painful aspects of being a man," says James Herzog, Ph.D., a training and supervising analyst at the nonprofit Boston Psychoanalytic Society and Institute and author of *Fathers and Play.* In fact, medical professionals in Australia suggested that many of men's mental health problems may stem from "the estrangement between fathers and sons...and the lack of self-worth this has created."

"If a man can't find a way to get what he so desperately seeks from his father—approval, support, acceptance, respect—no matter how much success he has achieved in his life, he ultimately will feel that he has failed as a man," Dr. Herzog says.

Song for My Father

She is the woman who smothers us with unconditional love. But he is the man whose love many men are never sure of. We look up to him. We look down on the world from his shoulders. Whether we adore him or abhor him, our father is our first and primary male role model.

Boys "turn to father because they have been conditioned to want a validation of their masculinity," sociologist Leonard Benson wrote in *Fatherhood: A Sociological Perspective*. Like the relationship between teacher and student or master and apprentice, he continued, father "serves as an exacting and insistent coach, acting out masculine patterns of aggressiveness. He drills his son continually, repeatedly calling attention to his mistakes.... Fathers crack down on their sons for failure to show signs of progress toward self-sufficiency."

This father-son boot camp basically conditions a son to strive to earn his father's respect, says Samuel Osherson, Ph.D., a psychologist at the Fielding Institute in Cambridge, Massachusetts, and author of *The Passions of Fatherhood* and *Wrestling with Love*. It also leaves us with a sense of insecurity, he adds, since it will take many years for us to perform as well as he. He keeps reminding us we're losers. So it becomes our mission in life to beat the old man at his own game. Since Dad is our model for what to expect from other men, we tend to generalize these reactions, to feel insecure around other men. We want their respect. We are determined to best other men. That is how we will win their respect.

But back to Dad. Now he has his own problems, says Ronald F. Levant, Ed.D., associate clinical professor of psychology in the department of psychiatry at Harvard Medical School and author of *Masculinity Reconstructed, Between Father and Child*, and other books

Members Only: The Men's Club

One way we earn our fathers' respect is to pass the initiation test that allows us VIP privileges at the club he belongs to—that would be the club of men. We call them rites of passage.

For the Samburu tribe of East Africa, it involves a young boy's painful and traumatic circumcision, witnessed by his male relatives. He must remain motionless and silent for the 4 minutes it takes to cut off the foreskin of his penis. So much as a twitch and he's "forever shamed as a coward and will be excluded from attaining full adult status," according to David Gilmore, Ph.D., professor of anthropology at Hunter College in New York City and the State University of New York at Stony Brook and author of *Manhood in the Making: Cultural Concepts of Masculinity*. Across the continent in West Africa, before the boys of the Mende tribe are considered men and can take a wife, the elders induct them into what's called the Poro Society by scarifying their bare backs with hooks or blunt razors. Sambia boys of New Guinea go through six initiation rites starting at age seven that span 10 years. Among the less savory tests, they must perform fellatio on an older man and ingest his semen, and have sharp grasses thrust up their nostril until the blood flows copiously.

"In many tribal cultures, it's the boy's biological father who administers the actual test," Dr. Gilmore says. The symbolic meaning of these ceremonial tests "clearly is about gaining acceptance from their biological fathers and the elder men of the community, both of whom are referred to as 'father,'" he adds.

about men. "He may be withholding respect from you because his father withheld respect from him," Dr. Levant says. "A son has to keep that in mind: Your father is doing the best he can with what he was given." Or wasn't.

And so it goes, the begats of disrespect, passed down from one generation of men to the next. So what's a son to do to break the cycle? Here's what the experts recommend to establish a healthier life with father.

Stop seeking respect. We already told you this father-son thing isn't easy, and here's proof: If you give up trying to earn your father's respect, odds are he will respect you for that. The reason, Dr. Levant says, is that he will realize that you've finally become a grown man able to stand on your own, no longer dependent on what he thinks. Call it the Zen approach to earning your father's respect. "The son has to do a little trick," adds Dr. Pittman. "He has to stop whining pathetically about how his father didn't love him enough—and then his father will love him more." In a way, he says, "the son has to act more maturely than his father, be more of a man."

Be honest about your disappointment. This is such a simple and obvious approach that many men don't try it. "Communicate to him that he and you are not seeing eye to eye, that you're not feeling comfortable about his judgment," suggests Dr. Osherson. "Just don't frame it as an accusation." Dad may be more responsive than you think. "As fathers get older, they are often interested in making peace, but they don't know how to start the conversation," says Dr. Osherson. So start it.

Show your appreciation. What a father most wants to know is that he has been a good father, that you still look up to him. So tell him. Tell him by sharing what you've learned from him about cars, how to wire a stereo, how to tip a waitress. Demonstrate it by doing well

what he taught you and letting him know who taught you to do it so well. "If a son can anoint his father in this way, the father can relax and, in turn, anoint his son with his respect," Dr. Pittman says.

Look in the mirror. It's entirely possible that the judgment you think is coming from your father is actually your own judgment of yourself.

Mother Your Mother

There's Mother's Day. There's her birthday. And then there are scant few other days of the year that you really demonstrate how much you respect your mother and show her how much you appreciated her doing your laundry, making your meals, reminding you that your father's birthday was coming up—and juggling her own responsibilities.

"Women want to be honored and acknowledged for doing a good job as a parent, but at least as much, they want to be valued as a person," says developmental psychologist Dr. Ann F. Caron. She contends that boys start to lose respect for their mothers when they sense their mothers backing down simply because their sons have gotten taller and sprouted muscles. That, in turn, triggers a chain reaction of mutual disrespect. To make it up to Mom, once you reach adulthood, reach out and make some of the following gestures—recommended by Dr. Caron—before reaching for a second helping of her outstanding strudel.

Take your mother to work. Introduce her to the people you work with, your boss, your secretary. Show her you are admired and respected and that you have grown up to be a fully responsible and mature adult.

Take her to lunch. Or buy her a cup of coffee. Get together with her on a one-to-one basis. Find out what she's up to, how the relatives are. Ask about her hopes, her dreams, her disappointments. "Indulge her," says Dr.

Caron. Let's not even count the number of hours she indulged you while you were (allegedly) growing up.

Thank her. **For helping you with your times tables. For being a one-woman Central Exchange, the conduit of communication for the whole family. For *not* telling your father about that bounced check. For instilling you with values that impressed the other wonderful woman in your life.**

Admit to screwups. **Remember that time right after college when you left for Canada in the middle of the night for six months without so much as a goodbye? Somehow you survived a cold war with each other for the next two years. Even if it's 10 years later, apologize for your immaturity. Tell her you realize how much that must have hurt her, showed her disrespect. It is never too late.**

Ask her to back off. **It's no coincidence that if you add an "s" to the beginning of "mother" you get "smother." They just can't help themselves. They knew you when you needed all the help you could get—feeding, diapering, burping. So when your mother keeps trying to burp you, metaphorically speaking, or meddle or pry or moralize or criticize or worry and try to "make it all better," politely let her know those services are no longer necessary. And you can move on together to a much more interesting adult relationship. Still, every now and then, just to let her know you still need her, bring your laundry for her to do.**

"When sons say their fathers criticize them for not being successful enough, not living in a big enough house, not whatever, I often see that it's about the son not being at peace with himself about those issues," Dr. Osherson says. "He hasn't lived up to his own expectation." Before you haul off on your dad for not giving you respect, do a gut check and ask yourself if you've earned your own respect. Accept your father for who he is—he's probably not going to change that much—and start working on yourself.

Listen to those war stories. Shower some focused attention on your father. "Listen to those old war stories he's been trying to tell you for a lifetime," suggests Dr. Levant. Get him to talk on his terms, not yours. Learn about his life. Ask him open-ended, nonthreatening, nonaccusatory, purely inquisitive questions about his relationship with his parents, his work, his old neighborhood. Show concern about his health, his plans for retirement. Spend time with him, with his friends, his bowling buddies. You'll see a side he doesn't know how to show you.

Act now. Reconciling whatever differences you have with your father may be tough, even painful. But one thing is for certain. It's nowhere near as painful as not doing it, Dr. Osherson says. "Too many men realize after it's too late that all they wanted to do was say, 'I love you' to their fathers," he says. "The man deserves your respect while he's still living."

Otherwise you'll carry to your grave the regret of missing the opportunity.

Become a father. Nothing will give you greater respect for your father than becoming one yourself. It's a gesture to your old man that you thought highly enough of his efforts to take a stab at it yourself, says Armin Brott, host of *Positive Parenting*, a radio talk show on KOIT in San Francisco, and author of *The New Father: A Dad's Guide to the First Year.* And it gives Dad a taste of immortality. Not only does he see his family genes projected into the future, but "having a child means your father gets to live his life over again through you," Brott says.

The Loving Husband

Respect:
The Real Love Connection

It even left Sigmund Freud, the father of psychoanalysis, scratching his scalp. "The great question that has never been answered," the Austrian pondered back in the early part of the twentieth century, "and which I have not yet been able to answer, despite my 30 years of research into the feminine soul, is, What does a woman want?"

Little could he have imagined that in the 1960s, the Queen of Soul would spell out and belt out the answer to his query. "R-E-S-P-E-C-T," Aretha Franklin sang. "Find out what it means to me." *Dat vazn't zo deefeecult, vazit, Herr Freud?*

Or was it? We have spent the last 40 years of the twentieth century trying to find out what that means to women as a gender. And more to the point, you have spent the last—what?—seven, 15, 25 years trying to figure out what that means to the one specific woman you promised you'd be with 'til death do you part.

He Said, She Said

Well, you're not to be blamed if you haven't exactly figured out where all the pieces fit in the Rubik's Cube of romance. If it's any solace—and we firmly believe confusion loves company—a survey conducted by Roper Starch Worldwide for the 1995 Virginia Slims Opinion Poll reflects

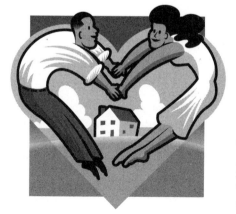

some seemingly contradictory trends regarding respect and marriage. Take a peek.

- On the one hand, 43 percent of women said their marriages had improved over the years, up 9 percent from 1990. On the other, the percent of women who said they were "very satisfied" with their relationships with their husbands or the men in their lives dropped from 56 percent in 1990 to 49 percent in 1995.
- While 74 percent of women and 73 percent of men agreed that men were more involved in their children's lives than they used to be, 48 percent of women resented the way child-care duties were shared and 47 percent resented the amount of time they spent keeping the family organized.
- Most women and men (81 and 80 percent, respectively) said that they admire a man who shows his sensitive side. But both women and men (84 and 85 percent, respectively) agreed that men were just as competitive as ever, and 57 percent of women and 43 percent of men thought men were still self-centered.
- While 72 percent of men said they had become more understanding of women's needs, only 61 percent of women agreed with that statement.
- In spite of 25 years of progress toward women being treated equally with men in society, 84 percent of women still believed that "regardless of changes that may have occurred, women still have more restriction in life than men do." And 77 percent of women said that "while sexual discrimination is more subtle and less open, it remains a serious problem today." Seventy-nine percent of women and 70 percent of men believed that some men still find it

hard to think of women as equals.

- There's a discrepancy about how much men are re-examining their behavior. While 70 percent of men said that women were too quick to call them sexist, only 57 percent of women thought that women were too quick to label men sexist. Also, 62 percent of men said that they were questioning their own macho roles, while 54 percent of women said that they believed men were.

- The bottom line is that 70 percent of both genders agree that "most men are confused about what women expect of them nowadays."

This brings us full circle to Sigmund Freud and Aretha.

What women want is for men to simply respect that being a woman is complicated and complex, a maze of mixed messages, suggests James Sniechowski, Ph.D., a Los Angeles–based counselor for men and co-author with his wife, Judith Sherven, Ph.D., of the book *The New Intimacy*.

"Men will earn women's respect more if they appreciate that no matter how far women have come since the women's movement of the 1960s, they are still raised to be second-class citizens and are still often treated that way," Dr. Sniechowski says. "Also, married women in their upper thirties, forties, and beyond struggle between wanting to be taken care of and wanting independence."

To earn their respect, he suggests, we need to not get caught in the backlash of their confusion. Sometimes we need to stand our ground, to hold it steady as she goes.

A Chore Thing

Sure, men are doing more housework these days, up from 20 percent of the work in 1965 to 34 percent in 1993, according to a study by Joseph H. Pleck, Ph.D., professor of human development and family studies at the University of Illinois in Urbana. But, as Dr. Pleck notes, "that's still far from the 50 percent that would represent equality." And, he adds, "there's something almost inherently disrespectful about the fact that men expect women to carry the brunt of the domestic responsibilities."

Even worse, women still get the most mundane tasks, says Rosalind C. Barnett, Ph.D., a senior scholar at Radcliffe College in Cambridge, Massachusetts, and co-author of *She Works, He Works*. Re-examining the data on chore-sharing, she found in a study that "female" tasks—planning and prepping meals, buying groceries, cleaning up after dinner, housecleaning, and doing laundry—were less under one's control. They were repetitive in nature and had to be done by a certain time and almost every day.

In contrast, many "male" tasks—making repairs around the house, taking out the garbage, doing yard work, and tending to the car—permit a higher degree of control. When you do them is more or less up to you. Low-control jobs, she found in her study, can be hazardous to your health. High-control jobs have little or no effect on your health. And, her study showed, the more time men and women spent doing low-control tasks, the lower they rated the quality of their marriages.

From all of this, Dr. Barnett suggests that—for the health of their wives, their marriages, and themselves—men should share the drudgery of some of those "female" chores. Figure out a schedule that allows you to do the onerous stuff on a rotating basis.

How Do You Spell Respect?

When it comes to keeping love alive in a long-term relationship, there is no issue more crucial than respect, says Scott Stanley, Ph.D., co-director of the Center for Marital and Family Studies at the University of Denver and co-author of *Fighting for Your Marriage.* "Over the years, I've seen that women have difficulty maintaining their attraction to men they've lost respect for," he says. "Men should never assume that just because they are married, they've earned that respect once and for all and go to pot, so to speak."

Preserving a lasting love, based on mutual respect, requires a certain vigilance. The garden won't flourish unless you keep watering it. Here are some ways to keep respect flowering in the garden of love.

Let her breathe. Despite the myth of men's inability to be intimate, "a lot of men feel intimacy has to be always, constant, and all-pervasive," says Mark Epstein, M.D., a psychiatrist in Manhattan and author of *Thoughts without a Thinker.* "That becomes claustrophobic." Many men today "have difficulty respecting the separateness or autonomy of the person they're involved with," he says. "They expect her to be catering to their every emotional need."

When she doesn't meet his needs, he pouts and withdraws or gets aggressive and even more demanding. Women have their own needs and identities that are not tied to the men in their lives, Dr. Epstein says. Men must learn to respect that. In other words, give her space.

Let her grow. She used to party hard. Now she's into meditation. Her idea of healthy eating once meant ordering a Big Mac because it had lettuce and pickles. Now she's dabbling with macrobiotics. Her values are changing, and

Arguing with Respect

Yes, women want men to listen to them. But they also want men to speak their minds. "Women respect men who don't shut down, withdraw, or pull away when issues come up," says the University of Denver's Dr. Scott Stanley. "That infuriates them."

The problem is that "what women call a discussion, men often call a fight," observes Diane Sollee, director of the Coalition for Marriage, Family, and Couples Education, a coalition based in Washington, D.C., that serves as a clearinghouse to promote education for couples. There's another problem.

As a means of self-preservation, husbands tend to "stonewall it" when they think women are trying to pick a fight, contends Daniel Goleman, Ph.D., a behavioral sciences writer for the *New York Times* and author of *Emotional Intelligence.* The reason is that it takes less emotional negativity for men than women to trigger the secretion of more adrenaline into their bloodstreams, which then increases their heart rates. "The stoic male imperturbability may represent a defense against feeling emotionally overwhelmed," Dr. Goleman says.

Dr. Stanley offers three quick tips for how to fight with your wife and still respect each other.

it scares you. You may be thinking that this is not the woman you said "I do" to. Welcome to the human species, friend. This is called evolution; it's called growing and changing, and it's supposed to happen to normal, healthy human beings. "We stereotype our wives," says Dr. Sniechowski. "After 20 years, we assume that she can't possibly say something that will surprise you." Surprise! Don't take her for granted, or she'll be out the door.

Embrace change. How many times

Separate the issues from the person. It's possible that the person you love may not like the same shade of purple that you love. She may even be a Democrat while you are a Republican. She says "po-tay-to," you say "po-tah-to."

But don't call the whole thing off. People are not their opinions. Assaults on people's personalities because they don't agree with your point of view are not fair and show no respect for the individual.

Avoid generalizations. "Always" and "never" are rarely accurate assessments of how frequently or infrequently people do things. "You always leave the cap off the toothpaste tube" may be true more times than not, but you are not giving your wife positive reinforcement for that one out of 10 times she remembers. And nine times out of 10 she will remind you of that time she did replace the cap.

Stay on point. Bringing up the time she met her old boyfriend for drinks while you're trying to argue about who forgot to close the car windows before a torrential rainstorm isn't fighting fair. Resolve one conflict at a time. Perhaps it's better to let sleeping dogs (and old boyfriends) lie, anyway.

remain open to new ideas.

Be your own man. Accept the fact that you can never be everything she wants. And she doesn't necessarily want you to be, either. "Many women are caught in a terrible bind," Dr. Sniechowski says. They're fighting off the idealized 1950s *Ozzie and Harriet* model they saw while growing up as well as the cynical 1990s version typified by *Married...with Children*.

If a man is too sensitive, he's a wimp. If he's not sensitive enough, he's a patriarchal troglodyte. What's a regular guy to be? Despite her wavering, "claim your own identity," Dr. Sniechowski says. That's what she wants and respects. Don't buckle under the pressure of every gender re-definition you read about in *USA Today*. Stick to your guns. She'll respect that more.

Drive on a two-way street. Dr. Sniechowski sees another ramification of the mixed messages that both sexes send each other. Men tell him, "She said she wanted me to share my vulnerabilities, but when I did, she freaked out and seemed to question my masculinity." Women can't have it both ways, he says. Dr. Sniechowski offers tough-love advice: "Demand it. Say, 'I will not *not* be human.' If the context is mutual respect, then as long as you are presenting her with who you are, she needs to accept that part of you, too."

Dr. Sniechowski says he and his wife, also a psychologist, resort to a caveat when they may not see eye-to-eye on how the other should behave. It goes like this: "I accept you exactly the way you are, *and* I reserve the right to want you to be different."

Take time. By now we know that women want to talk, want to be listened to, want to be heard. But that takes time. As much as you'd love to sit and gab, there's stuff that

has a buddy come to you with that sad, confused, clueless look in his eyes telling you that it came from out of left field when she left him, claiming she had outgrown him? You want to say, "What did you expect? How long did you think she'd be patient while you kept reading *Success* magazine after she had subscribed to *Simple Living*?" What you should say to yourself is, "Thank God it wasn't me." And promise yourself that you'll stay in tune with your partner's changing interests and needs to get done, lawns to mow, calls to the West Coast to return, and other manly responsibilities. Strike a compromise. All talks don't have to be intense, suggests Dr. Stanley. Spend 10 minutes here, 10 minutes there. "But make them a powerful 10 minutes," he recommends. Don't keep glancing over at the game on the tube while pretending to give her your full attention. "Even these short spurts are longer than some couples allow themselves," he says, and they serve as short-term pressure-reducers until longer blocks of time can be scheduled.

Play ball. Of course, those longer periods have to be scheduled. They don't just materialize magically, says Dr. Stanley. And, he suggests, agree as to whether you'll be discussing heavy issues or just enjoying playtime. If you opt for play—and even adults deserve recess—agree not to discuss the mundane, nagging details of your shared life ("Did you call the refrigerator repairman?" "Have you finished the financial aid forms for Junior?"). Save that for a business meeting in which you clear the deck of all domestic duties.

Cut out the cutting remarks. Little put-downs show clear disrespect. Those negative comments can do more to corrode a relationship than positive efforts can do to keep it strong and vibrant, Dr. Stanley warns. He particularly singles out the man who cuts down his wife in the company of other people. "This is a guy who doesn't have the *cojones* to tell her in private," he says. "He has been chewing on something for a while and doesn't have the guts to tell her more respectfully in private, so he does it in the safer context where he knows she's not going to make a scene in front of friends or family."

Surviving Infidelity

Adultery happens, perhaps more often than you think. A study conducted by the National Opinion Research Center reported that 21 percent of men and 13 percent of women admitted having had an affair at some point in their lives.

"We're not such a monogamous species as people would like to believe," says Harriet Lerner, Ph.D., a clinical psychologist in Topeka, Kansas, and author of *The Dance of Deception* and *Life Preservers*. "Affairs are not terrible aberrations that happen only in terrible marriages."

Though Dr. Lerner asserts that there are no etched-in-stone strategies and techniques for winning back respect after an affair, she offers several guidelines.

Tell her before she finds out. If you confess the affair before she discovers it, you'll at least earn some leniency points.

Do some soul-searching. That affair may be the tip of a glacier-size iceberg of marital unhappiness. Maybe you want out of the marriage and this is your way of making that painfully clear. If you don't want to stay married, lying about wanting to stay married adds insult to injury. "Continuing the deception is showing disrespect for her and yourself," says Dr. Lerner.

Commit to the process. If you want to remain married, be prepared for many conversations over time. "Be

His advice to men like this is to grow up. "Get up the gumption to say that you'd like to discuss something that has been bothering you. But don't bring it up when it happens. Try to discuss it when you're not emotionally charged, when you're both in a supportive and loving mood." Then she'll understand that you're trying to respect the ready to sit in the hot seat," Dr. Lerner says. Don't expect that one confession, regardless of how heartfelt it is, will regain her trust.

Give her time...and space. Tell her that you understand it will take however long it will take her to make sense of and recover from this break of trust. Say, "All I can tell you is how committed I am to not letting this happen again." Say this only if you mean it.

Avoid false promises. Don't say, "I'll never be tempted to wander again." Even in the best of marriages, people are attracted to other people, Dr. Lerner says. "We are all tempted. Perpetuating a lie or keeping an attraction secret can only corrode the relationship even more."

Don't volunteer details. Be open to any of her questions, but don't confess more than you need to, suggests Dr. Lerner. Months or years later, when she feels safely distant from it, she may ask. Then tell her.

Use this as a wake-up call. "People get sleepy about their marriages, and a great deal of distance can get entrenched," Dr. Lerner says. "When someone has an affair, the other spouse suddenly pays attention." An affair does not necessarily signal the end of a relationship, the end of trust and respect. "I've seen marriages strengthen and deepen after the revelation of an affair," she says. "It's a call for a deeper commitment to truth."

Ph.D., associate professor of gerontology and psychiatry at Virginia Commonwealth University in Richmond. Dr. Dougherty was part of a team that examined why some couples successfully go the distance. Marital satisfaction, they found in couples married an average of 22 years, was directly related to how "outgoing, warm, positive, gregarious, and ebullient" the partners were. Wives said the more kind, considerate, and thoughtful their husbands were, the higher they rated the quality of their marriages.

"This is common sense," she admits. "People like being around people who are nice to them, have a positive outlook on life, and like and are liked by other people." But Dr. Dougherty puts another spin on this obvious wisdom. Outgoing people focus on others, she notes. We all like having that attention focused on us; it makes us feel special, respected. (This would be especially true of women who feel that they are still not valued as first-class citizens.) People who were more self-centered, she found in other studies, did not have happy marriages.

Be willing to work at it. Just because your life together isn't going as smoothly as a greeting card doesn't mean that you're doing something wrong. "It's not simple," Dr. Sniechowski says. "Love is full of ambivalence and ambiguity. If it's rocky, you haven't made a mistake. In fact, you may be doing something right." That certainly is the case if you're venturing into deeper emotional waters. There's going to be a period where you're afraid that you're in over your head. But working through those times together will bring you closer and lead to a deeper, more satisfying relationship.

integrity of the relationship. If you continue to use sarcasm and cynicism and put-downs as your primary communications strategy, it's time to consult a professional, such as a therapist or psychologist, for help, according to Dr. Stanley.

Be a happy hubby. Happy people have happier marriages, says Linda Dougherty,

The Wise Father

Being There for Your Children

In the beginning, earning your children's respect is as simple as a hug and a ride on your shoulders.

"Your kids worship you," says Lawrence Kutner, Ph.D., a psychologist who is on the faculty at Harvard Medical School and the author of *Your School-Age Child* and *Making Sense of Your Teenager.* "You are huge, powerful, and brilliant."

That lasts until they reach puberty. Then fasten your safety belt, secure your ego, and prepare for the full frontal attack to your position of authority. (For more about teenagers, see The Patient Father of Teenagers on page 107.)

Meanwhile, according to Wade Horn, Ph.D., president of the National Fatherhood Initiative in Gaithersburg, Maryland, whoever said that 90 percent of life is just showing up could also have been talking about fathering—good fathering, that is. But even that's not enough.

"Fathers earn their children's respect and have a positive impact on their development not only by being present but also by being involved," Dr. Horn says. "Our research shows that when fathers are engaged in their children's lives, their children have greater self-esteem, perform better in school, exhibit a more secure gender identity, and generally have greater success in life," he says. And he backs that statement up with some evidence.

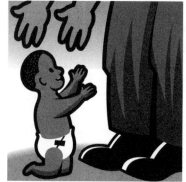

- Premature infants whose fathers spent more time playing with them demonstrated better thinking and reasoning skills at age three.

- A survey of African-American men revealed that men who had experienced a positive relationship with a father who cared and sacrificed for them are more likely to be responsible fathers themselves.

- A survey of 455 students ages 14 to 19 found that those with higher self-esteem and lower depression reported having greater intimacy with their fathers.

Don't Be a Stranger

Despite what seems to be clear evidence that fathers play a key role in the development of children, many are still missing in action, whether the excuse is divorce, the obligations of work, or the awkwardness that comes with tackling an unfamiliar role. Chew on some of these raw data.

- When 1,500 chief executive officers and human resource directors were asked how much leave is reasonable for a father to take after the birth of a child, 63 percent indicated "none."

- According to a 1996 Gallup poll, 79 percent of Americans feel "the most significant family or social problem facing America is the physical absence of the father from the home." Four years earlier, 70 percent felt that way.

- The number of children living only with their mothers grew from 5.1 million in 1960 to 16.3 million in 1994.

In the Trobriand Islands east of New Guinea, anthropologist Bronislaw Malinowski found that the name given to fathers was *tomakava,* which translates to "outsider" or "stranger."

That gives a whole new meaning to the saying, "Don't be a stranger." And fathers would do well to follow that advice, says David Popenoe, Ph.D., associate dean of the faculty of arts and sciences at Rutgers University in New Brunswick, New Jersey, and author of *Life without Father*.

Whether you are a single father or just a distracted dad, he says, "the single most important thing is regular contact, spending time together, showing your children you care deeply and will be there."

Show them *and* tell them. "Make sure that your children know you love them," he says, "and the most direct way is to verbally tell them so." For single fathers, Dr. Popenoe warns, "Don't be a Disneyland Dad."

That's the father who takes his kids on weekends and spoils them with 48 hours of ice cream, movies, and, yes, trips to Disneyland in lieu of what they really want—attention.

"Play a part in their daily lives," Dr. Popenoe suggests. "And if you have them only weekends, help them with homework, make dinner together, sit around the living room doing nothing—but doing it *together*." A lot more goes on—a lot more respect is earned and connection made—in that downtime together than you'd suspect.

Dad, the Disciplinarian

To be sure, earning your child's respect is an uphill battle. "There has been a significant erosion of parental authority in the last 15 to 20 years," says Laurence Steinberg, Ph.D., professor of psychology at Temple University in Philadelphia and author of *You and Your Adolescent*.

Saying You're Sorry

In his maudlin 1970 bestseller *Love Story*, Yale University professor Erich Segal coined the catchphrase, "Love means never having to say you're sorry." That's a lot of bunk, particularly when it comes to children, says psychologist Dr. Lawrence Kutner of Harvard Medical School.

"No one is perfect," says Dr. Kutner. "If you present yourself as perfect, your child will see himself as a failure. The key to maintaining his respect and your integrity is to apologize. You'll be surprised at how remarkably forgiving kids are."

What do you do if you snap at your kids? Dr. Kutner suggests:

- Apologize without excuses. **Not apologizing "sends the message that your behavior was okay," Dr. Kutner says. So admit it: You screwed up. Let your child know that you overreacted because things were tough at work. But make sure you add, "That's no excuse for showing you disrespect."**

- Apologize without excusing them. **If your mistake was triggered by theirs, make sure they hear that what they did or said or didn't do or didn't say was not appropriate behavior.**

- Resist bribing them. **Don't add, "What can I do to make it up to you?" Offering to take them to a movie or buy them ice cream or a toy only serves as reinforcement for them to repeat whatever it was that ticked you off in the first place.**

- Be a role model. **Showing them you are "man enough" to apologize gives your children permission to do the same thing when their turn comes.**

- Learn from it. **Let your child know that you will *try* not to let it happen again. That, too, models behavior that shows you're both on a learning curve as parent and child—and that, as humans, you both may screw up again.**

- Don't overdo it. **It terrifies a child when her parents keep apologizing. "They start to assume you're unpredictable and unstable," Dr. Kutner says.**

Regrettably, he notes, some men figure that taking back authority—and thereby earning respect—means being a tough disciplinarian.

"The drill sergeant is one extreme, and it clearly doesn't work," says Dr. Kutner. But being too lenient and indulgent neither earns respect nor teaches a child about appropriate limits.

"The most effective parents are loving but also demanding," adds Dr. Steinberg. "They treat their children's interests and problems as meaningful and at the same time set well-defined limits that they enforce strictly and consistently." Dr. Steinberg offers some specific guidelines on how to command respect without coming off like Sergeant Carter (even when your kid acts like Gomer Pyle).

Explain the rules. When parents are willing to discuss the rules and regulations, taking time to explain why they have to insist on this or forbid that behavior, children are less likely to rebel. You can start this at very early ages so that by the time they are teenagers, you'll have less of a rebellion.

Distinguish between punishment and consequence. A punishment is something a parent does to you. A consequence is something you do to yourself. "Punishment is one of the least effective ways of getting your child to cooperate," Dr. Steinberg says. When a child connects the consequences of spilling milk to mopping it up, he will more likely be careful the next time.

Let them set the consequence. Ask your children what they think they should do as a consequence of their misbehavior. Parents often find that children impose much stricter penalties on themselves than the parents themselves would.

Know what's nonnegotiable. Rules that cover physical and emotional safety and deeply held family values should not be open to discussion or debate.

"You need to know where and when to draw the line," says Dr. Steinberg. "Children will respect that."

Here are some other suggestions for fathers, culled from other experts.

Be a less-than-Super Dad. Too many fathers think they earn their children's respect by playing the role with a big S on their chests, impressing with their competence at and knowledge of everything. That doesn't inspire respect; it inspires an inferiority complex, warns psychiatrist and family therapist Dr. Frank Pittman III.

"The ideal father sometimes acts like a bumbling idiot to lower the bar for his child," he says in a surprising twist on the typical advice to be a bigger-than-life role model. "Let your kid feel more heroic. Don't overwhelm him with your power and masculinity. That's the sign of an insecure parent."

Pay attention. When your child interrupts you while you're on the phone or trying to finish some project, "that's often a call for attention," says Armin Brott, host of *Positive Parenting*, a radio talk show on KOIT in San Francisco. Sometimes, it's the only way a child can say, "Hey, what about me?"

Make the most of playtime. Kids pick up a lot of messages at playtime, says Ross Parke, Ph.D., professor of psychology and director of the Center for Family Study at the University of California at Riverside and author of *Fatherhood*. And so do psychologists. "We see important implications for social development in the play patterns between father and child," Dr. Parke says.

Children who said that they enjoyed playtime with their fathers adapted to playing with other children better than those who disliked playing with Dad.

And what determined how much they enjoyed pushing those Legos around with Pop? "The most successful dads read their child's nonverbal cues" and adjusted their own behavior according to the child's mood, says Dr. Parke.

The Patient Father of Teenagers

Understanding the Awkwardness of Adolescence

"What are you doing?"

"Nothin'."

"Where are you going?"

"Nowhere."

"Whom are you going with?"

"No one."

If this sounds like the rich and informative repartee you and your offspring have been having lately, welcome to the parents' equivalent of the Twilight Zone. Welcome to your child's teen years.

"How does a teenager spell individual? R-E-B-E-L." That spelling lesson is offered by Jane Nelsen, Ed.D., president of Positive Discipline Associates in Sacramento, California, and co-author of *Positive Discipline for Teenagers.* "It's the teen's job to find out who he or she is," Dr. Nelsen says. "This could mean testing your power."

Could?

To earn their teenager's respect, parents need to understand that child development is like manifest destiny. In order to get from the East Coast shores of childhood to the West Coast of adulthood, young people have to cross the Great Plains of adolescence. The best we can do during these turbulent years is to "keep our perspective," says Dr. Nelsen.

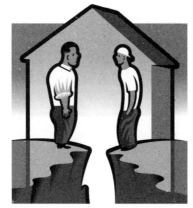

Respect Is Letting Go

"The adolescent doesn't want you to solve his or her problems anymore," says Temple University's Dr. Laurence Steinberg, author of *You and Your Adolescent*, which he based on a three-year study of adolescent behavior and attitudes. He tries to allay parents' concerns about this much-feared period: "Relax! The horror stories you have heard about adolescence are false." He found that almost nine out of 10 teens do not get in trouble with drugs, delinquency, or irresponsible sex.

On the other hand, he says, "when parents expect the worst from their adolescent, they often get it." Fail to respect them, and they will return the sentiment—in spades. He adds, "When parents show respect for their teenager's point of view, are willing to discuss rules and regulations, and explain why they have to insist on this or forbid that, the adolescent is much less likely to rebel."

Knowing what to expect at each stage of development, Dr. Steinberg notes, "is half the battle." So let's start by defining the terms we'll use throughout this chapter. The rule of thumb is that preteens are ages 10 to 12, teenagers are 13 to 17, and young adults are 18 to 21.

But, Dr. Steinberg adds, adolescents develop at different rates. So if your 11-year-old son is already blasting power chords on his Fender Stratocaster guitar and sprouting little hairs on his face, you can assume he's a little ahead of the game. And you should adjust your game plan accordingly.

Meanwhile, it may help you to know that while you're trying to earn his respect, he's struggling to get some of his own from his peers. Two-thirds of teens participating in a Yale University study said their school was noisy, and more than half said students disobeyed rules. Only 24 percent felt that students respected each other, and only 31 percent said that they helped each other.

The Parent Traps

The cornerstone of mutual respect is that you can count on each other's word. Once you've both agreed on a deadline for a chore or any other commitment, it's important that your teenager (and you) honor that agreement. Even so, "I can almost guarantee that if your teen promised to do the lawn by 4:00 P.M., it will not be done," says Dr. Nelsen. But here's where the fun and games begin. When your teen says he's ready to split for the mall at 4:00 P.M. and the lawn still looks like a rain forest, ask, "What was our agreement?" No matter what excuse he has or plea bargaining he attempts, stick to the contract: "What was our agreement?" Dr. Nelsen promises that 90 percent of the time, they will succumb if you just keep repeating that phrase.

Letting teens break an agreement is one of the four traps Dr. Nelsen identifies that defeat respectful parenting. The other three are:

- Believing your agenda is theirs. Mowing the lawn is on your Top Three list of things that need to get done this weekend. It's not in your teen's Top 100. "Believing that something that is important to you is important to your teen sets you up for disappointment," Dr. Nelsen says.
- Getting into put-downs. Do you remember how insecure you were as a teenager? Self-doubt is a mantra that follows teenagers from the moment they look in the mirror in the morning until the moment they look at

"Dad, Did You Ever Do Drugs?"

When President Bill Clinton confessed that he had tried marijuana—but didn't inhale—he merely admitted he was a member in good standing of a generation that felt obliged to push the envelope on alternative lifestyles. Now the tables are turned and you're trying to be a pillar of respectability for your teen, who's eager to test the edges himself or herself. Do you tell the truth and set a bad example? Do you lie and set another bad example? What *do* you do if your kid asks whether you did drugs?

"I definitely don't think it's a good idea to lie," says Lloyd Johnston, Ph.D., program director of the Monitoring the Future research project and senior research scientist at the Institute of Social Research at the University of Michigan in Ann Arbor. "Eventually, your kids find out everything about you anyway. Then everything else that you say to them will have no credibility."

He believes there is nothing hypocritical about asking your children not to do what you did. "I wouldn't offer information until I was asked," he recommends. "It's not necessary to spill your guts. Try starting a conversation by asking what other kids think about drugs. Indicate that as a parent you hope they stay away."

If they ask if you've tried drugs, and you did, then say yes. When they say, "See, you tried it and you're okay," Dr. Johnston suggests using some of these arguments to explain why it's not such a great idea for them.

We were young and naive. Just because we did something then doesn't mean we still think it's a good idea. We knew a whole lot less about the consequences of taking

themselves before they go to sleep (and the hundred times they look at themselves in the mirror in between). No need for you to exacerbate the situation.

drugs in the 1960s than we do now. For example, experts said cocaine use was not addictive. That turned out to be grossly incorrect.

The drugs are stronger now. That designer weed they're cultivating nowadays packs a lot more wallop than it did back then.

Kids are trying drugs at much younger ages. We were in college when we tried it. Studies show that marijuana use had tripled from 6 percent in 1991 to 18 percent in 1996 for eighth graders; it more than doubled from 15 percent in 1992 to 34 percent in 1996 for 10th graders; and it jumped from 22 percent in 1992 to 36 percent in 1996 for high school seniors. "We find that the earlier they start, the more trouble they tend to have with other problems," Dr. Johnston says.

There's higher risk all the way around. In many ways, we live in a more complicated—and dangerous—world than 30 years ago. For one thing, we didn't have the threat of AIDS, and research shows that people take more sexual risks—like not using condoms—when they are high on drugs.

For more information on how to talk to your kids about drugs, write to Growing Up Drug-Free, Pueblo, Colorado 81009 for a free copy of the brochure "Growing Up Drug-Free." Other sources of supportive information include the National Clearinghouse for Alcohol and Drug Information, P.O. Box 2345, Rockville, Maryland 20852; and the Partnership for a Drug-Free America, 405 Lexington Avenue, New York, New York 10174.

Have you tried confidence-building compliments? Surely, your teens must be doing something right. "Where did we get the idea that in order to encourage kids to do better, we have to make them feel worse?" asks Dr. Nelsen.

• Not sticking to the issue. When the goal is to get them to mop up the sticky soda they just spilled all over the kitchen floor, there's no need to bring up every other example of klutziness they've displayed in the last 72 hours. It's definitely not the right time to bring up that incomplete they're looking at for not finishing the chemistry project. Take it one issue at a time.

A Parenting Primer

As you and your teen attempt to cross the Great Plains of adolescence with mutual respect intact, it might help to keep Mark Twain's recollection in mind: "When I was a boy of 14, my father was so ignorant I could hardly stand to have the old man around. But when I got to be 21, I was astonished at how much he had learned in seven years."

Here's a primer to help parents get through those seven years.

Respect their privacy. This is a hot button for young adults, says Barbara Lynn Taylor, a trainer and lecturer on parenting skills based in Winston-Salem, North Carolina, who is the author and producer of "Successful Parenting," a video-based parenting series. Their bodies are changing almost every day, and that embarrasses and confuses them. And they don't want you to see what's going on. So don't burst into their bedroom or the bathroom if the door is closed. Knock. After all, you expect the same.

They're also beginning to develop a life of their own that they value very highly. It's their first step into real independence. So don't go through their backpacks or their mail. "Parents have to let go of the idea that their kids are their possessions and they have a right to invade their children's private areas," Dr. Nelsen says. The same is true for one of the most private—and scariest—places in teenagers' lives: their minds. If there's something they don't want to discuss, "don't grill them on what they're thinking," Dr. Nelsen says. "They will only retreat further."

Increase their responsibilities. If you give them the key to the car when they come of age without first entrusting them with smaller responsibilities, you're looking at a very stressful evening for both you and your child. "Trust is part of a continuum," Taylor says. "Build it up at an early age and by the time they're teenagers, you won't be locking horns over the biggies."

Back off on public displays of affection. Don't be hurt if the son who held your hand in public now makes you feel like a leper when you're together at the mall. "They want to be loved and want to know you love them—but not in front of anyone who they might know...or anyone they might not know," Taylor says. In private you can joke about this with them, but in public respect their need to put so-called childish things behind them. Later in life they'll come back to hugging and kissing.

Have a dialogue, not a monologue. "Too often parents want to talk to their teens and not with them," Dr. Nelsen says. We lecture in the name of education but, she points out, the Latin root of educate means "to draw forth."

"We try to stuff wisdom into them, and then we think they're being disrespectful when they don't respond to this inappropriate style," Dr. Nelsen says. Try a conversation in which you ask more questions than you offer answers.

The Birds and the Bees

A father goes to his son and says, "It's time we talked about the birds and the bees." The son replies, "What would you like to know?"

That today's teenagers are more sophisticated about sex than we give them credit for is both true and false, says Temple University's Dr. Laurence Steinberg, author of *You and Your Adolescent*. It's true that by the time they graduate from high school, about two-thirds of them will have engaged in sexual intercourse. But they still operate with a lot of false assumptions about birth control, contraception, and how infectious diseases are spread, for example. And that may be our fault. A Harris Poll found that two out of three teenagers have never talked with their parents about birth control. But when asked how they would choose to learn about sex, nine out of 10 say from their parents, according to Dr. Steinberg's study.

"The goal is to teach them to make decisions for themselves," says Barbara Lynn Taylor, author and producer of "Successful Parenting," a video-based parenting series. "And we need to trust them to make them."

Granted, talking about sex could be one of the most awkward conversations you'll ever have with your child. But it doesn't have to be. Try these approaches.

Pick a comfortable time. If you feel uneasy about

For instance, ask them what they learned from an experience and how they might do things differently.

The goal is to encourage teens to willingly open up about themselves. There's a big payoff. In his study of 20,000 teenagers, Dr. Steinberg found that teens who share the details of their lives with their parents are less likely to have trouble with their schoolwork or to get involved with drugs and alcohol.

having the conversation, make it easier on yourself and your child by finding a time when you don't feel work stress or time constraints, Taylor says.

Be straightforward. In fact, the birds and bees approach is outdated, says Dr. Steinberg. Explain the "facts of life" not as an analogy or parable but in clear and plain English, being specific about what goes where, how, and when. This does not have to be a lecture in human anatomy. But be prepared to answer such questions as, "What's a vulva?" Use clinical words. The vocabulary of sexuality is charged, so use terms such as sexual intercourse instead of its slang euphemisms, and penis and vagina instead of...you get the picture.

Be patient but persistent. If they literally get up and walk, too embarrassed to allow you to continue, don't press them. But try again, perhaps this time in a letter, stating the basics or suggesting a book or video. Reassert that you understand it may be difficult to talk about the subject but that you're available whenever he or she feels more comfortable.

"It's important that your child understand that having the discussion is important to you and that you tried," adds Dr. Steinberg. "That alone is comforting for a teenager." If you can't get across to them, encourage them to talk to someone such as a guidance counselor, aunt, or uncle.

family outing, maybe they get to see the concert this year but commit to attending next year's soiree. If the group performs again sometime soon, maybe your child joins the family but gets to go to the gig the next time. "Look for the win-win," says Dr. Nelsen. And she suggests that you, being the wiser and more mature person, closely examine how attached you are to getting your way just to assert your authority.

Can the clichés. Clichés don't work because they are like elevator music. Kids have heard these lines for so long that they—heard this cliché?—go in one ear and out the other. They have no meaning, no clout, no credibility, and certainly no creativity. Here are some that carry absolutely no weight with teenagers (or people of other ages) and, in parentheses, what teens are probably saying to themselves in response.

"Go to your room and think about what you just did." (*"Sure, if I can find time to fit it in between e-mailing my girlfriend about what jerks you are and figuring out how not to get caught the next time."*)

"You think the world owes you a living?" (*"No, just enough money to get me on a plane to Hawaii and away from you."*)

"I'm not your maid." (*"Well, if you were, I'd fire you for doing such a lousy job.*)

Brainstorm solutions. Here's a remedy to the teenager's frequently justified complaint that decisions are made for, not with, them.

Say, for example, you'd like them to attend the family picnic, but they want to attend a concert. Have a joint problem-solving meeting. The agenda is: How can we both get what we want? (Big clue: One of you may have to delay gratification.) If it's an annual

Limit the lecture. The only person listening to your lecture is you. "Kids tune out as soon as they even hear that lecture tone of voice," Dr. Nelsen says. After about the fifth word, they're on another planet—where parents have mutated into small throwaway plastic dolls. Instead, try one-word reminders. "Dishes." "Lawn." "Homework." If you're extremely verbose, add a second word: "Please."

The Respectful Son-in-Law

When Her Family Becomes Your Family

They are, for the most part, human lottery numbers that come at no extra charge with the person you marry. Some of us get lucky and draw the most wonderful in-laws extant. Others, well, don't.

"In-laws are almost like the people you work with at the office," says Gloria Call Horsley, a family therapist in San Francisco. "You didn't pick them, but you have to live with them and make it work."

Getting your wife's family to show you some respect—forget about ever getting them to bless their lucky stars that she married you and not that millionaire Beverly Hills plastic surgeon she was dating—is going to make your life much more enjoyable. Trust us on this. But it's not going to be easy.

Remember that saying, "A daughter is a daughter all of her life; a son is a son until he takes a wife"? One of the implications is that when a man marries, he inherits two more parents. And therein lies a very big problem, according to Emily Martinsen, a therapist dealing with family systems who practices in Ocala, Florida, and author of *The Troublesome Triangle: Son, Wife, Mother-in-Law.*

"Men often see their mothers-in-law as their mothers, and just as they did with their mothers, they feel the need to pull away so that they don't get smothered or turned into puppets," Martinsen says. Pulling away does not ingratiate

you to your new mom. Or, by association, your new dad.

Naturally, earning their respect starts with showing them respect. And there's a residual benefit to doing so. "Showing respect for your in-laws shows respect for your spouse," Martinsen says. So you're earning extra points on the home front.

You'll earn the most respect from your in-laws "by respecting them as individuals and respecting them individually," says Horsley. So first of all, don't assume your mother-in-law is just like your mother and your father-in-law is a spitting image of your dad. And erase all those mother-in-law clichés, jokes, and other stereotypes from your memory (and your repertoire).

Then, suggests Horsley, "don't lump them together as a unit. Get to know what they're like separately. Find out about their personal interests." And take interest in those interests. Ask "Dad" to show you that stamp collection, and then buy him a rare first printing. Offer to take "Mom" to the flower show, and buy her some seeds. That kind of thing.

The Nine Lives of In-Laws

To help us get a fix on their uniqueness, Horsley has eliminated the guesswork by detailing in her book *The In-Law Survival Manual* the nine "types" of in-laws and the best strategies for gaining the respect of each. So put on your best son-in-law sweater (the one her mother gave you for your birthday) and take some notes.

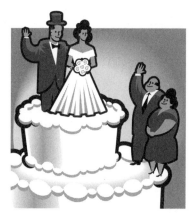

1. The critical in-laws. These are the ones who always think you could have a better job, a nicer suit, a more expensive house—or at least one that's closer to them. They tend to expect you to be prompt and to do what you say you'll do. So try to be on time, and live up to promises and commitments. Since this type is so comfortable being direct, if you're angry with

them, confront them in person—but in private. They'll probably admire you the more for your straightforward approach.

2. The giving in-laws. These in-laws give until it hurts—time, money, homemade lasagna, a shoulder to cry on, an ear to complain to. But they want the same in return. So give it. Acknowledge their kindness and largesse by taking laser-focused interest in them. Or they'll turn a cold shoulder to you.

3. The super-achieving in-laws. These in-laws have a to-do list the length of an orangutan's arm and try to impress you with how successful they are. A classic Type A personality, they often end up super-extended and stressed out. Let them know you like them for who they are and not just for what they've achieved. Gently remind them when you think they're working too hard, and invite them to do something relaxing with you (if they can fit you onto their to-do list).

4. The emotionally intense in-laws. Among the most high-energy people on the planet, they have the capacity for great depth of feeling. Also called drama kings and queens, they have no qualms about telling you their "real" feelings. Life with them is a roller coaster: their lows as low as their highs are high. Appreciate the fact that they feel strongly about life. Accept their mood swings. If you see them going down with their dark side, encourage them to lighten up; try to show them the bright side of things. Take them to a comedy club.

5. The observant in-laws. These are the relatives who sit on the sidelines, watching the action but rarely jumping in on family conversations or activities. They may appear shy but actually just enjoy the more contemplative perspective. Respect their choice to watch rather than participate. Honor that they are enjoying it all in their own style. But because they tend to be overlooked, every now and then take a moment to go over and give them a hug or throw a knowing smile or wink their way. That gesture will be most appreciated—if not reciprocated in some demonstrative way.

6. The opposing-view in-laws. They love to argue strictly for argument's sake. Nothing personal, mind you. But they are hypersensitive to slights. If you do cross the line into personal criticism, they will hold a grudge for the longest time. If you like a heated debate, you're in for a mutually thrilling relationship. Just remember the rules: Don't make fun; don't let the debate turn to personal attacks; separate the person from his or her ideas—and let them win every now and then.

7. The gadabout in-laws. They're always on the go, always with somewhere better to go. You should not be surprised if they call Saturday night to cancel out on the Sunday brunch you invited them to weeks ago because they were invited on their neighbors' yacht. Don't let their flurry of activities fluster you. Forgive them for their flightiness. If a social engagement you've invited them to is a top priority, make sure they know—they will be there (especially if you happen to mention Donald Trump may be dropping by).

8. The take-charge in-laws. They are the overbearing bosses who also have the ability to pull together the whole family for reunions. To deal with them, practice saying this statement first to yourself: "I'm feeling uncomfortable with the way you often take over." Then approach them privately and say it out loud. If they really rub you the wrong way (which may be due to the fact that you, too, are a take-charge person), excuse yourself from the decision-making process. If that doesn't work, excuse yourself from the room.

9. The conflict-avoidance in-laws. Every family has one: the Solomon who can see all sides, is a good listener, good advice-giver, good secret-keeper. But while they're busy solving everyone else's problems, their own are starting to make Mount Everest look like a molehill. Because they tend to be overlooked, you may win friends by sharing information, asking their opinions, following through on their suggestions. Make them feel as though someone's concerned about their problems by showing you can play a fairly decent Solomon yourself.

The Loyal Brother

Moving from Rivalry to Respect

There's a wonderful Peanuts cartoon in which Lucy, the domineering big sister, is watching TV. Behind her is her little brother Linus, sucking his thumb, his ubiquitous security blanket clutched to his cheek. "You are my younger brother and I am your older sister," she says. "And that's the way it's going to be all the days of your life...." Then she adds, "And don't tell me you never think about it," which sends Linus into a twitching scowl.

We enter the family stage, it often seems, already typecast. We're the oldest, the middle, the baby. A chip off the old block. The apple of Mom's eye. The whiz kid, the do-gooder, the klutz, the comedian, the troublemaker. The ham, the shy one, the moody one.

"Many of us were assigned roles in our families, often relating to how we fit in with our siblings," says Jane Greer, Ph.D., a psychotherapist in Manhattan and author of *How Could You Do This to Me?: Learning to Trust after Betrayal* and *Adult Sibling Rivalry: Understanding the Legacy of Childhood.* "These childhood roles become restrictive, even suffocating."

When we continue to see each other in those same roles—the brother who Mom liked more, the sister who always bossed you around—we are not honoring the fact that they (and we) have changed. That's disrespectful.

Furthermore, siblings overpersonalize conflicts with each other, contends Frank Sulloway, Ph.D., a research scholar in the science, technology, and society program at the Massachusetts Institute of Technology in Cambridge and author of *Born to Rebel: Birth Order, Family Dynamics, and Creative Lives.* "I believe they would show greater respect for each other by understanding the extent to which their behaviors are reflections of genetic patterning that go back thousands of years," he says.

After reading and analyzing close to 30,000 biographies, Dr. Sulloway concluded that birth order may be one of the most important factors in determining a person's personality. His basic premise is that older siblings tend to be controlling, adhere to traditional values, and support the status quo. Later-borns are more open-minded, more innovative in their thinking, the rebels of the family.

"Birth order turned out to be the single best predictor of attitudes toward radical innovation," Dr. Sulloway says. So when your big brother or little sister starts acting out, cut them some slack: They're only reading from a very old script.

He Ain't Heavy, He's My Brother

We're not just talking about young brothers and sisters who show each other disrespect. Childhood competitiveness follows siblings into adulthood. In one study, 71 percent of subjects ages 21 to 93 said they had been rivalrous with a brother or sister. Of those, 45 percent admitted those feelings persisted. (By the way, half of that 45 percent said those feelings were precipitated by parents favoring one sibling over the other. So to you parents out there, *stop playing favorites.*)

Meanwhile, as somebody's brother, you can end the family feud and earn respect in a number of ways. Try these tips.

Draw the line. When your sibling crosses the line,

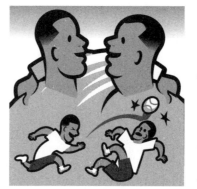

you'd earn respect—and save yourself discomfort—by just saying no. Here are some examples of crossing the line: Your brother borrows a lot of money for the umpteenth time. Your sister interrupts you at work to complain for a half-hour about Mom and Dad. Your oldest sister harangues you to "get your life together" (when hers is falling apart at the seams). How do you know where and when to set the limit? "When it feels intolerable, when what they do makes you angry or makes you feel guilty, when it makes you feel very uncomfortable—that's going over the limit," Dr. Greer says.

Move on with your life. Old slights, lingering cold wars, past disappointments: It's easy to hold on to these. "It takes an active stance and trust to move away from them," says Dr. Greer. Try saying, "Let's agree to leave the past in the past. Let's start anew."

"You have to agree on this," Dr. Greer says. "Even the clunkiest verbal attempt at this is better than silence."

Ask for advice from your older sibling. They feel it's their birthright to know more about everything than you. So pay them their propers. "It's no skin off your chin to build their ego," Dr. Sulloway says.

Pull together. Siblings pull together when there's little or no competition for parental favor, Dr. Sulloway found. For example, this may happen if both parents are poor or so distracted by their own worries and concerns that they pay little attention to the children. "Nothing brings siblings together faster than a family emergency, a death, or an accident," he says. Suddenly, holding a grudge against your brother for stealing your G.I. Joe when you were 10 has very little relevance. So why is it relevant now? Don't wait for tragedy to bury the hatchet.

Find a niche. Competing within the family for the same area of expertise only creates conflict and reduces your chances of emerging as the family expert on any given subject. If your older sibling is already the family comic, become the king of the kitchen. Dr. Sulloway's favorite example of this is Ralph Nader, the consumer advocate, each of whose brothers and sisters selected a separate specialty in life. All went on to great things—and more important, all maintained great rivalry-free and respectful relationships with each other while benefiting from each other's knowledge.

Oh, Brother!

While older siblings tend to be controlling and adhere to traditional values, younger siblings are more open-minded and rebellious, according to the Massachusetts Institute of Technology's Dr. Frank Sulloway. Here are two men who changed the world because of the order in which their mothers changed their diapers.

Benjamin Franklin. A youngest son, Franklin was indentured at the age of 12 to his elder brother, a printer. "My brother...had often beaten me, which I took extremely amiss," he later wrote. At 17, he escaped his brother's control by moving to Philadelphia. Publisher, scientist, statesman, kite-flier, Franklin was an innovator to the core.

Charles Darwin. It was examining Darwin's life that led Dr. Sulloway to investigate the effect of birth order on one's life in the first place. Darwin wrote of his older brother: "Our mind and tastes were so different that I do not think that I owed much to him intellectually—nor to my four sisters." He wrote that his father once said to him, "You care for nothing but shooting, dogs, and rat-catching, and you will be a disgrace to yourself and all your family." Not to Dr. Sulloway's surprise, Darwin went on to offer one of the most bold and radical innovations of all time: the theory of evolution.

The Good Neighbor

Respecting Privacy and Possessions

Thank God for the definitive rule on how to earn respect from your neighbor. The dilemma of this difficult relationship was anticipated early on, so He sent Welcome Wagon's first representative, a man named Moses, back to the 'hood with a basket containing an even 10 commandments. One of them went a little something like this:

"You shall not covet your neighbor's house; you shall not covet your neighbor's wife or his male servant or his female servant or his ox or his donkey or anything that belongs to your neighbor."

But since it wasn't specifically mentioned, many men interpret that to mean we *can* covet our neighbor's 25-horsepower, six-blade, five-speed Toro lawnmower. Right? And, alas, since no mention was made relating to the statute of limitations on how long you can borrow said power mower before said neighbor loses respect for you, you assume that you can keep the mower 'til the (golden) calves come home. Right?

Wrong.

Reaching Out

Actually, there's nothing all that complicated about being a good neighbor. The best way to earn respect from the folks next door is to respect their possessions and their privacy.

"People value their privacy," says Susan Gross, national vice-president for Wel-

come Wagon, a greeting and advertising company that was established in 1928 to introduce newcomers to local businesses. Today there are more than 2,500 representatives in 5,000 cities knocking on newcomers' doors with their familiar welcome basket. "Good neighbors respect and honor each other's right to privacy."

At the same time, Gross adds, "people have a deep need to reach out to each other, and they want to be reached out to." Especially with new neighbors, she says, "I advocate making that first gesture, just to let people know you're there if they need anything or want to know where to shop for groceries, hardware, whatever. You don't have to see each other every day for the rest of your life."

In this mobile society—about 17 percent of the American population moves in a year, according to the U.S. Census Bureau—many people live far from where they grew up, "so the neighborhood becomes your extended family," says Marian Montgomery Leck, manager of an award-winning Neighborhood Watch program in The Woodlands, a community of approximately 48,000 people about 27 miles north of Houston. The group, whose goal is "to create a sense of community and a safe community," promotes neighbors relying on neighbors to recognize unusual activity on their streets and to know when to call the local police.

"Neighborhood Watch is not peering into someone's window," Leck says. "It's ownership of your street and making sure everybody is okay. Taking responsibility for each other shows and earns respect."

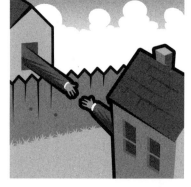

Building Good Fences

Other than rereading The 10 Commandments, there are a number of ways to endear yourself to your neighbors. All of the following demonstrate that you respect your neighborhood, which, in turn, demonstrates that you respect your neighbors, which, in turn, will earn you their respect. Let us count the ways.

Cover for each other. If you notice your neighbor left his garage door open when he left for work, or his apartment door ajar, call him and ask if you should close it (if you have his work number). Otherwise, close it for him—unless you think there's a possibility he left it open on purpose. If you know your neighbors are away on vacation and you see their mail and newspapers stacking up—always an open invitation for burglars—take it in for them, suggests David Rechenmacher, public affairs manager and director of the police community support division for the village of Downers Grove, which is 25 miles west of Chicago. Better yet, if you know before they're going, offer to do it for them if they don't ask. As a gesture of trust and faith, consider asking them to take yours in when you split town.

Keep it up. Your property, that is. Fix that drain. Repair the shingles. Paint the house. Mow the lawn for gosh sakes—after all, you've had your neighbor's mower since the summer of 1995. Keeping your home in top shape improves the look of the neighborhood, adding to the value of your neighbor's home as well as your own. That way, you can both hold each other in highest respect sitting side-by-side poolside in retirement on the French Riviera.

Sit on your front porch. Be a part of National Night Out, suggests Leck, whose Woodlands community has won awards for its participation in the nationwide event that occurs on the first Tuesday of August. The theme is "giving crime and drugs a going-away party." At neighborhood block parties, games and contests for kids, adults, and seniors are geared around issues of public safety to "build bridges between the police department and the neighborhoods," says Leck. The event encourages people to hang out on their front porches

TV Neighbors

In all the known universe there is one breed of man who cannot survive without a neighbor: the TV sitcom star.

The legacy passes from Art Carney's Ed Norton on *The Honeymooners*; to the well-meaning neighbor *and* landlord Fred Mertz in *I Love Lucy*, played by William Frawley; to Archie Bunker's worst nightmare come true, a Black neighbor named George Jefferson, played by Sherman Hemsley; to the one-and-only oddball Kramer in *Seinfeld*, played by Michael Richards. All are barely tolerated, occasionally appreciated, infrequently respected, and even more infrequently respectful of their neighbor, even if he is the star of the show.

"You love them or you hate them," Alex McNeil, author of *Total Television*, says of TV neighbors. "And just like TV scriptwriters need neighbors to play the foil or the confidant to the stars, we need them to give us a sense of community, of belonging."

and get to know each other, and to leave their front porch light on all night. "The whole event helps break down the 'us' versus 'them' mentality," Leck says.

Host the first barbecue. Especially if you've won ribbons for your hot Texas-style barbecue sauce. You'll earn respect for making the first friendly gesture—and then can sit back and watch all the invitations come in for future get-togethers.

Build a backyard fence. American poet Robert Frost was right: "Good fences make good neighbors." But in American suburbs, it's best to limit your fence-building to the backyard, says Gross. Build one around your entire property, and people will think you're some kind of elitist isolationist snob—or you're building a bomb behind it.

The Trustworthy Friend

*Regular Guys,
Doing Stuff Together*

Clichés are clichés because people overuse them, not because they aren't accurate. We can't think of a better way to sum up this chapter than with this old saw: Make new friends but keep the old; one is silver and the other gold. Or, to pitch the notion from a higher plane, as it says in the Apocryphal Book of Ecclesiasticus (9:10): "Forsake not an old friend; for the new is not comparable to him: a new friend is as new wine; when it is old, thou shalt drink it with pleasure."

And now there's social science research to confirm all of this. According to a study by Rosemary Blieszner, Ph.D., a gerontologist at Virginia Polytechnic Institute and State University in Blacksburg and co-author of *Adult Friendship*, old friends were rated higher on a "love" scale than new. New friends scored higher on a "like" measure. "For young people," she says, "the message is: Keep your old friends."

Their value is twofold. For one, Dr. Blieszner found that older people with long-term balanced friendships were happier than older people with friendships of unequal power. Also, friendships are good for your health. They may even prolong your life. Several studies have shown that people with the strongest social and community ties were the least likely to die. The most isolated people had the highest death rate. In a five-year study of heart disease patients, those with neither a spouse nor a friend were three times more likely to die than those involved in a caring relationship, according to Redford B. Williams, M.D., professor of psychiatry and director of the Behavioral Medicine Research Center at Duke University Medical Center in Durham, North Carolina.

Side by Side

Among the greatest male myths is that men don't have old friends or new, that we don't know how to make or be friends, don't have respect for the institution of friendship, don't concern ourselves with earning other men's respect, that we stonewall our way through friendships that appear as cardboard-thin as Marlboro man billboards, revealing little of a deeply personal nature about ourselves, and that women have more and better friendships than we do.

That might have been how it looked from the surface, but new research shows that men and women "just have different styles of friendships," says Jan Yager, Ph.D., a sociologist and workshop leader based in Stamford, Connecticut, and author of *Friendshifts: The Power of Friendship and How It Shapes Our Lives*. Her book, published in 1997, is based on surveys and/or interviews with several hundred men and women throughout the United States and several other countries.

"From an early age, boys' friendships with other boys are more competitive and activity-oriented than same-sex friendships between girls or opposite-sex friendships," Dr. Yager says. "Men are traditionally taught to be more private and to avoid revealing anything about themselves that might hamper their rise up the corporate ladder. Until recently, the only area in which men felt comfortable revealing much about themselves was with their wives or, if unmarried, with their romantic partner, their

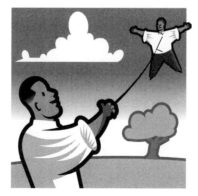

clergyman, or their therapist." But, she notes, this is changing—men today are more likely to open up to their friends than men of the past.

But the fact is that men crave the respect of other men. "Friends are the mirrors that reaffirm our self-esteem as men," says Scott Swain, Ph.D., a sociologist who has published papers on male friendship and is currently a counselor at Las Lomas High School in Walnut Creek, California. We just express our friendship in different ways. We have what psychologists call side-by-side relationships; women have face-to-face relationships. In other words, we show our closeness by doing stuff together. Women do it by sitting across from each other, talking directly to each other.

People have an average of one or two best friends, four to six close friends, and 10 to 20 casual friends, Dr. Yager found. But there were some surprising results in terms of what she found about men and friendship. Men, she reports, had twice as many casual friends at work as women. Her explanation: "To be successful, you have to get the whole company to like you. The loner doesn't make it in the corporate world." Another surprise: While men complain that they don't have many friends, that may be because "men have a higher standard of what a friend is," concludes Dr. Yager. "Women are quicker to include more levels of friends. Men don't consider casual bowling buddies as friends." But when you break it down, she adds, men and women have about the same number of friends.

Being a Buddy

So what's holding us back from making new friends and better cherishing our old buddies? Good

Finding Old Friends

You were neighborhood chums back in White Plains, or drinking buddies in Ann Arbor, or foxhole buddies in Nam, or bookin' buds at law school. Then you got a job on the other coast, got married, got kids, got way too serious for your own good. And you've lost touch with the one guy in the world who can make you laugh simply by singing the opening lines to the University of Michigan fight song.

Join the club. That's the pattern, says Donald Pannen, Ph.D., executive director of the Western Psychological Association in Tacoma, Washington, who has studied the changing nature of friendships. "It's usually nothing dramatic that ends a friendship," he says. "People take different tracks. You move away, get busy raising a family."

Younger men cite these reasons more than older men, he has observed, probably because we go through more changes in our youth. But, he adds, women are better at maintaining friendships that meant something to them. And, he adds, men should get better at it.

"Old friends are the keepers of your shared memories," he says. "They help you understand that your life is part of a continuum."

If you want to play Sherlock yourself, here are *Men's Health* magazine's five favorite Web sites for tracking down people (all start with http://www.).

- People Finder at peoplesite.com
- World Alumni Net at alumni.net
- Switchboard at switchboard.com
- Bigfoot at bigfoot.com
- Global Mega-People Finder at trendy.net/sites/peoplefind

question. And here, respectfully submitted by our experts, are some even better answers.

Open up slowly. "You don't have to spill your guts to be a friend," says Dr. Yager. "Men need to learn to carefully reveal intimacies in stages." That's for two reasons. One is for himself: The practice of talking about one's most personal concerns with another man may not feel all that comfortable. The other is for your friend: You don't want to bowl this person over with more information about you than he or she would feel comfortable knowing.

Give it time. It takes about three years for two people to become tried-and-true friends, Dr. Yager found. "Be aware of this trying-out period," she suggests. During that time, there will be shifts in your personal life; see if your friendship weathers those changes. This phase also helps you see how much you can trust this friend. Share a less important small secret and see if it's kept or blabbed.

Look for reciprocity. Friendships don't develop if one person feels he's giving and it's not returned, says Dr. Blieszner. "Human beings seek balance in relationships. It doesn't work if it's one-sided." Ask yourself, "Am I just taking or just giving?" If you keep inviting your friend to do things and he or she isn't asking you out, you may be giving more than you're getting. It may be a subtle message that the other party is not that interested in a friendship with you. Stop asking that person to get together. Let him ask you for a change. If he never does, that's a not-so-subtle message. Invest the energy in another friendship.

Sidestep the competitiveness. There will always be the friend who loves to remind you that his RV is bigger than your RV—or his whatever is bigger than your whatever. "Don't buy into it—it's an illusion," recommends counseling psychotherapist Marvin Allen, director of the Texas Men's Institute in Austin and author of *Angry Men, Passive Men*. "These friends are looking for respect in all the wrong places."

So how do you steer clear of the natural male-style competitive banter without coming off as a stick in the mud? Here's Allen's strategy:

"I'll say, 'Wow, that *is* a big Winnebago.' And then I'll bring up something of a more personal nature. Like, 'That will be great to go out alone with your son, eh?'" The point is to show that you appreciate his great big RV but that there is something about him that is far more deserving of respect.

Ask for accountability. In plain English, we'd say: Call each other on your stuff. It's called accountability in the language of Promise Keepers, the international Christian outreach program with headquarters in Denver that hosts stadium conferences, educational seminars, and local church meetings. "We talk about taking responsibility for one's own actions and inviting other men to do the same," says Rod Cooper, Ph.D., a counseling clinical psychologist who is the organization's former national director of educational ministries. "If I don't draw your attention to things I believe you could do better in your life and you do the same with me, we think we will live happily ever after." That could not be further from the truth, he says. Sometimes you have to make waves with each other to show how much you care. "Have the guts to break the code of silence as a demonstration of your concern for him, and it will blow him away," he adds.

Befriend a woman. This is easier said than done. If you saw the 1989 film *When Harry Met Sally*, with Meg Ryan and Billy Crystal, you may have identified with Crystal's character, who summarized the difficulty of sex-free male-female friendship this way: "No man can be friends with a woman he finds attractive. He always wants to have sex with her. Sex is always out there. Friendship is ultimately doomed, and that is the end of the story." Not so, says Dr. Yager. She found younger boys are now developing more opposite-sex friendships than in the past—perhaps the younger generation is leading the way in the next age of sexual equality. In addition, she also noted, with more women in the workplace, men are seeking more friendships with women that do not include a sexual agenda.

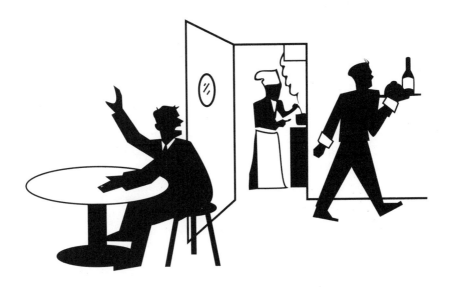

Part Five

Respect Wherever You Go

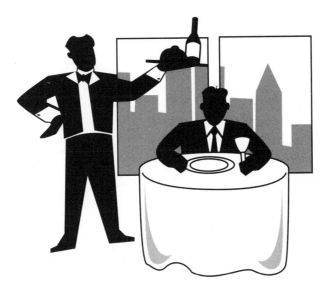

Dealing with Professionals

How to Score a Power Tie

They have letters after their names. You don't. They have impressive-looking bronzed diplomas from prestigious institutions of higher learning hanging behind their desk. You don't. They make big bucks. You...well...don't.

Even if your response to all of the above is "So do I," it still seems as though professionals—doctors, lawyers, dentists, accountants, and other white-collar business types—have an edge over us when we sit across from them for an appointment. They shouldn't.

"Society has put these people up on a pedestal," says psychologist Warren Farrell, Ph.D., author of *The Myth of Male Power.* "Then we resent them for it. In effect, we're jealous and intimidated. We shouldn't be. They just happen to know some things we don't. But we know some things they don't."

Among the professionals who are often able to intimidate us, to make us feel at least a tad unworthy, are lawyers, because they hold the keys to the legal system; accountants, because they hold our wallets in their hands; dentists, because they hold our delicate jaws in their hands; and doctors, because they hold our lives in their hands. We asked experts working in these fields how to garner their respect. Here's what they told us.

Courting Lawyers

First off, they've heard them all. And winced. So save the litany of lawyer jokes, like,

"What's 40,000 lawyers at the bottom of the ocean? A good start." (Sorry, we couldn't resist.)

"Lawyers want to be treated with respect, but not reverence," says Judge Michael Obus, justice of the Supreme Court of the State of New York for the County of New York and a former attorney with the Legal Aid Society of Nassau County, New York.

To save yourself time and, therefore, money, he suggests preparing for a court appearance or an interview with a lawyer by being able to discuss all pertinent aspects of the case, and by listening carefully to the questions and providing clear answers.

Now here's the hard part, Judge Obus adds: "You must overcome the lack of trust that is necessarily the case, particularly in a criminal case, when you view your lawyer as part of the system that is prosecuting you. You're only making that attorney work harder to prove not only his or her competence but also their interest in defending you."

Leo Stoller, executive director of Americans for the Enforcement of Attorney Ethics, a nonprofit organization that offers procedural advice for dealing with less-than-scrupulous lawyers, offers for starters a more pragmatic tip: "The number one way to get respect from an attorney is to put everything in writing." That's *everything.*

"Lawyers spend their whole life reading," Stoller says. "It's the medium they most respect and best respond to." And, in case of any disagreements (read: legal malpractice action you may have to take against your own lawyer), there's a paper trail.

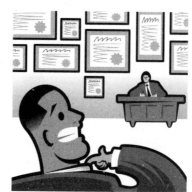

As soon as you're considering retaining an attorney, send him a letter, rather than calling, explaining exactly why you are seeking his services. If you decide to retain him, get a written retainer agreement that establishes an attorney-client relationship. Write "attorney retainer" on the check you send.

Keep a log of any phone calls between yourself and your lawyer. Don't use a tape recorder. Attorneys won't talk to you if they know you're using one. And unless they know, it's illegal to record your conversations with them. You should realize that when they put you on a speakerphone, they usually have a witness in the room. You should do the same.

Theresa Meehan Rudy, program director for HALT—An Organization of Americans for Legal Reform, a Washington, D.C., nonprofit group, adds several good suggestions.

Interview several attorneys. Let the attorney know from the outset that you're planning to meet with a number of lawyers to determine who would best handle your case. Learn what they might charge, how they plan to structure the payment, how they plan to handle the case. Ascertain if there will be a charge for the initial meeting.

Find an expert. Hire a lawyer with expertise in the area of the law that addresses your problem, not a generalist. Otherwise, you'll end up paying extra money on the time the lawyer will have to spend learning that area of the law, Rudy says. Ask these key questions: "How many other cases like this have you handled? What were the outcomes? What would be the first couple of steps you'd take in this case?"

Manage your case. Let counsel know that you intend to carefully manage your case. Make it clear that you're not turning it over entirely, that you plan to remain interested and active. This puts them on notice that you want them to be communicative with you, Rudy says. This is a common problem. Attorneys like to see themselves as professionals, not service providers. They sometimes forget who is working for whom.

Your Day in Court

So you finally have your attorney's respect. Now you're standing in the middle of a courtroom, looking up at a person draped in black and sitting above you behind an impressive desk. Meet the judge, the legal system's King Solomon. New York Supreme Court Judge Michael Obus offers free counsel on how you can get respect from a judge.

Speak or write in simple terms. Too many people think they have to write or speak in flowery, overly formal terms or legalese. "They think it will help their case," Judge Obus says. "It won't." What helps is direct, clear language—plain English. Profane language can earn you contempt—which, in court, carries jail time.

Dress appropriately. That means tie and jacket, or suit. "That demonstrates you show respect for the court," Judge Obus says. He advises wearing nice clothes, especially on the day a decision is to be made.

Bring a lawyer. Don't think that going it alone will earn you more respect. Just the opposite. And coming with an attorney "will make your life a lot easier," says Judge Obus. A lawyer knows the procedures and protocols that will expedite matters. In a criminal case, "it would be foolish to appear without counsel," he adds.

Accounting for Accountants

There's nothing sexy about number crunching. In fact, it's downright boring. But these are the men and women who make your work *work*.

"You have to think of it this way," says Michael Mares, partner with Witt, Mares, and Company, a firm of certified public accountants in Newport News, Virginia, and chairman of the tax executive committee of the American Institute of Certified Public Accountants. "I have an expertise that you're going to capitalize on. I work for you."

Here are several ways to keep the respect ledger balanced between you and your accountant.

Set goals. You don't have to be financially successful to impress an accountant at the outset of your relationship. "But I want to see that you have a game plan, goals, and a time frame in which you expect to achieve greater financial success," says Jack Lapidos, president of Geyer, Lapidos, and Van Horn, a San Francisco accounting firm that has been specializing in individuals and small businesses since 1974.

Some of his clients started as "starving artists"; now at least they are not starving. "I respect someone who says, 'I love what I do and I believe in myself.' I admire people who remake themselves."

Organize your life. Or at least your receipts. Lapidos offers three tips for organizing tax receipts.

- Have three types of back-up data. Those would be canceled checks, credit card bills, and receipts and copies of receipts for cash payouts.
- Keep receipts and other back-up data at least three years. That's how far back the IRS will look if you're ever audited.
- Break down all the back-up data into categories: office equipment, travel, entertainment, and so on. Total each category and give the accountant only the totals.

Share your secrets. Revealing the intimate financial details of your business operation is like opening the drawer where you keep your dirty laundry. No one blames you for feeling a little vulnerable when you're opening

---

Surviving an IRS Audit

It's the threat that intimidates more than the actual audit. Like you were caught cheating (even if you were innocent). And now the principal has called you in to pronounce your punishment.

Staring down an Internal Revenue Service auditor, his plastic pen holder placed properly in his shirt pocket, is an exercise in humility. Here are several tactics to minimize the effect.

Assume you're innocent. "The taxpayer should not think we suspect him of being dishonest," says Joan Schafer, IRS spokeswoman for the Pennsylvania District of the IRS in Philadelphia. Your name was either randomly selected or was chosen based on what the IRS calls your DFS score (Differential Function System), which means something about your return tripped a computer warning light. "So try not to come in with a defensive chip on your shoulder," adds Schafer.

Comply first, complain later. Your audit notification will tell which records are being requested and which to bring. Bring them. Once you've shown up for your meeting,

---

your books to a professional. "You have to trust your accountant and be honest," Mares says. "In our profession, confidentiality is paramount. I cannot help you or advise you unless you're honest."

That means not withholding facts to get the kind of answer you think your accountant wants to hear. He will respect you less—not more—for that.

Respect the limits of the law. Have a good sense of what may be deductible and what may not. Your accountant will let you know if it counts or not. Lapidos suggests applying what he calls the sleep test. If you lose sleep over whether it's tax-deductible, it probably isn't. Don't declare it.

then ask for an explanation regarding why those records are being requested.

Present all receipts in an organized fashion. If you bring in a shoebox full of receipts and have no idea how to find the travel and entertainment receipts for which you're being audited, the auditor will not respect you—and will probably look at your return with that much more suspicion. Organize them. Label them. If it's entertainment expenses that are being questioned, on each receipt note the name of the business associate you dined with and what you were meeting about.

Take it up with a higher authority. If you feel that the auditor has not given you a fair hearing, you can request an immediate meeting with an examiner supervisor to explain your position, Schafer says. Still no satisfaction? Write to the IRS District Director or Service Center Supervisor.

Keep the faith. You may think it's a losing battle, but the IRS reports that of the 2.1 million audits in 1995, 78,404 taxpayers and corporations got a grand total of $2.8 billion back.

Know the Drill with Dentists

First they make you wait big-time in the waiting room, force you to read *National Geographic* magazines from 1959, and torture you by piping in easy listening covers of The Rolling Stones. Then they make you wait in the chair. Finally, you are rewarded for all your patience by having pain inflicted on you.

Want respect from your dentist? Start by spitting out that 1950s version of your relationship with your dentist, advises Christine Dumas, D.D.S., assistant professor of clinical dentistry at the University of Southern California in Los Angeles and consumer advisor for the American Dental Association.

If that is the way your dentist treats you, make a quick retreat from that office. "It should be a comfortable, pain-free, and positive experience," says Dr. Dumas, who has a dental practice in Marina Del Ray, California. "Dentistry used to be a passive experience for the patient. You went. They did things to you. Six months later you went back. Today we see it as a partnership. You're with your teeth a lot more than I am. There are things I'll ask you to do between visits. The question isn't how to get respect from your dentist; it's how to get you to respect your own teeth."

Meanwhile, Dr. Dumas suggests improving your relationship with your dentist by sinking your teeth into the following tips.

Schedule an early appointment. If you want to beat the waiting game, come as early in the day as possible, before the delays start compounding. Also, the first appointment right after lunch break is a safe bet. Ask your dentist's office manager to give you a call at your office to advise you of any delays. In turn, Dr. Dumas says, a respectful patient won't cancel at the last minute or be late for an appointment himself.

Meet the manager. A dentist hires an office manager as a reflection of himself or herself. If you like the manager, chances may be good that you'll like the dentist. But this should not take the place of meeting the dentist.

Get the dentist to say "Ah." Well, not quite. But do interview the dentist. Word-of-mouth recommendation is one way to find a dentist, but it may not be the best way. Make sure you feel comfortable with this person who will be spending a lot of time with his or her fingers in your mouth. Ask if he or she is on the faculty at a teaching institute or is a member of the American Dental Association. It's also a good idea to ask if the office staff is required to take continuing education courses (in dental-related fields, of course).

A Prescription for Dealing with Doctors

There's something about that white coat. Or maybe it's knowing how much they spent to get through medical school. Or how much you're going to spend to get out of their office. Whatever it is, doctors intimidate simply by virtue of being doctors.

"Doctors have a lot of training and knowledge, and we respect that," says Timothy McCall, M.D., staff physician at St. Elizabeth's Medical Center in Cambridge, Massachusetts, and author of *Examining Your Doctor.* "It's like, who are we to second-guess a doctor?"

The catch-22 of getting respect from doctors is that we usually go to see them when we're not feeling well, when we are not feeling at the top of our game. "It's well-known that when people become seriously ill, they regress," Dr. McCall says. "We're seeing them when they're feeling most vulnerable, when all they want is to be taken care of."

To establish yourself on more equal footing with a physician, he suggests going to your appointment armed with as much information as possible about what you think is ailing you. Reliable sources are the national associations and organizations that provide free information on various diseases. (See "Health Information Services.") Then ask questions to fill in the blanks of what you don't know or understand. This will impress your doctor. It may even force your doctor to go beyond what he or she knows. At the least, it will make your doctor explain things to you rather than just prescribe medications. Aside from following some of the same advice you just read about dealing with dentists, here are some other pre-

Health Information Services

These national organizations are a good place to start when you want free pamphlets, brochures, referrals to support groups, and other information about a number of leading diseases.

American Cancer Society
1599 Clifton Road NE
Atlanta, GA
30329-4251

American Heart Association
7272 Greenville Avenue
Dallas, TX
75231-4596

American Lung Association
1740 Broadway, Floor 15
New York, NY
10019-4374

American Psychological Association
750 First Street, NE
Washington, DC
20002-4242

scriptions for getting respect from a doctor.

Check your doctor's ears. You want a doctor who listens to your explanations and problems. If the doctor interrupts before you feel you've sufficiently explained the situation and ailments, your respect alarm should start ringing, Dr. McCall says. According to a survey of malpractice attorneys, more than 80 percent of their suits are due, in part, to poor doctor-patient communications. One study shows that doctors who've never had any malpractice claims tend to have longer visits with patients

Asthma and Allergy Foundation of America
1125 Fifteenth Street, NW, Suite 502
Washington, DC
20005

National Diabetes Information Clearinghouse
1 Information Way
Bethesda, MD
20892-3560

National Headache Foundation
428 West St. James Place, Second Floor
Chicago, IL
60614

National Health Information Center
P.O. Box 1133
Washington, DC
20013

National Organization for Rare Disorders
P.O. Box 8923
New Fairfield, CT
06812

Get it in Latin and in plain English. Doctors often explain what you're suffering from solely in lay language. "The impulse is good," Dr. McCall says. But when you only have a lay explanation, you can't go look it up. You can't discuss it with another doctor.

Get a second opinion. Speaking of speaking to another doctor, Dr. McCall says it would not show disrespect to a physician to say you'd like a second opinion. "Trusting physicians implicitly is a dangerous proposition," he says. In situations that might require aggressive treatment, like surgery, "it's becoming standard practice to get a second opinion," he notes. "If your doctor does take umbrage, that's not a good sign that this person has your best health in mind." Telling your physician that you plan to have another doctor examine you is more than a professional courtesy; it may save you money and hassles if tests you've already had done—and paid for—can be forwarded to the second doc.

React naturally. People respond to news of their medical condition in various ways. Many worry that their reactions are being monitored and judged by their physicians. Some are stoic—because they think they'll get more respect. Others break down—because they think they'll get more respect.

and routinely ask more questions about their patients' medical problems and treatments than doctors who've had two or more malpractice claims against them.

Listen really carefully. Assuming the doctor does his or her part, you, in turn, have to do yours. Listen. If you have a mind like a sieve, take notes. If that's too distracting, ask permission to tape-record parts of the appointment in which the doctor is explaining or prescribing. Alternately, bring a friend or family member who can listen or write for you.

"Good doctors don't care," says David Loxterkamp, M.D., a family practitioner from Searsport, Maine, who is on staff at Waldo County General Hospital in Belfast, Maine, and author of *A Measure of My Days: The Journal of a Country Doctor.* "We give patients permission to be whomever they need to be at that moment. You lose no respect for getting angry, frustrated, for crying, or any other human reaction. We've seen it all and accept it all."

In a Restaurant

How to Get Served with a Smile

In the 1991 film *L.A. Story*, comedian Steve Martin offered his depiction of what it sometimes feels like to get a restaurant reservation. The competition is so fierce and the pretension so thick in Tinseltown that his character is forced to suffer through a grilling from his banker before the maître d' of a certain snooty eatery will book a table for him.

Martin once again may have let his imagination run a little too wild and crazy. But he certainly struck a familiar chord with many restaurant-goers. "Many Americans feel insecure and intimidated because they're put on the defensive by people in the restaurant business who forget that the customer is always right," says Eric Asimov, who writes the "$25 and under" restaurant reviews for the *New York Times*. "The customer's typical response is either meek submission or overbearing belligerence."

Neither may be the best response if you want to get a little respect—and a lot of service. But if you're one of the people who contributes to the $104 billion spent annually in America's 177,000 full-service restaurants (those with waiters and waitresses), you've probably reacted that way at least once with one of the 9.5 million employees within the industry.

Respect without Reservations

Eating out is practically an American way of life. The typical American consumed an average of 4.1 commercially prepared meals a week in 1996,

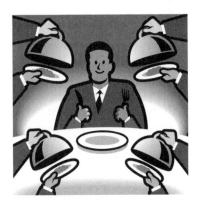

according to the National Restaurant Association. Men eat out more than women: 21.8 percent of the time for men compared to 18.1 percent for women. And guys ages 18 to 24 eat out nearly six times a week. With that many opportunities to win or lose respect, we figured the following tips would be more useful than a *Zagat* restaurant guide.

Pick a restaurant that's appropriate. "The restaurant you pick tells the person you've invited how much respect you have for them," says Philip Smith, who teaches operations management at the New England Culinary Institute in Montpelier, Vermont. If you don't know much about the local restaurants, check local newspaper reviews or skim through a regional restaurant guidebook or the trusty old *Zagat*, which includes customers' comments, both pro and con.

Ask for special treatment. If you're celebrating an anniversary, birthday, or contract signing with an important client, ask for the manager when you're making the reservation. Tell him or her you want them to pour it on with the VIP treatment. Ask for a chilled bottle of wine or champagne to be waiting when you arrive. Maybe they'll prepare a special dessert cake with an inscription on it. "You don't have to give the person a $10 bill beforehand," notes Smith. This all implies you know what good service is—and how to reward it at the appropriate time (if you don't, see page 130).

Be on time. Only one thing will earn you less respect than being extremely late for a reservation (without a legitimate excuse), says Giuseppe Pezzotti, a lecturer in food and beverage management at Cornell University's prestigious School of Hotel Administration in Ithaca, New York. "That's what they call in the trade a no-show." If you're stuck in traffic and going to be late, call ahead (one good argument for a car phone). If you have to cancel, call. That's called courtesy. It may allow the establishment to go ahead and book your table. It may also keep your name off the mud list and assure you a seating the next time you call to book a table.

Show interest. "As soon as we know someone is excited to dine with us, all our alarms go off," says Brenda Thompson, manager at The Fountain at the Four Seasons Philadelphia, which was named one of the top 25 American restaurants by *Food and Wine* magazine and the Top Table in Philadelphia by readers of *Gourmet* magazine. "After all, we're in this business to serve *you.* Taking us for granted may be the biggest disrespect you can show us." Ask about specials. Ask about ingredients, where they come from, how they're made. If you sound interested enough, you may even be honored with a thank-you visit at your table from the chef.

Talk the talk. Let the staff know that you understand their business by using words specific to their industry, suggests Eric Weiss, founder and president of Service Arts and a Manhattan-based consultant specializing in service issues. Like this: "I know your expediter must be up to his ears in orders, but could you please check on our dinners?" Expediters are the ones who announce the orders once they come into the kitchen, and they sometimes put the final touches on the plates before they go out to the dining room.

Don't make a scene. If it seems like hours have passed since you last saw your waiter, don't snap your fingers and shout "garçon." That is annoying and disrespectful, says Pezzotti. Rotate your head looking to make eye contact with anyone who looks like they work there. If

Respect in the Fast Food Lane

Every meal out cannot be a Michelin Three Star event. There's not enough time. Or money. That's why man invented fast food. The operative word is fast. "Okay, so we're not a candlelit dinner," says Kevin McNamara, director of worldwide operations training for Burger King's over 8,000 international restaurants. Still, you should expect a satisfactory experience when you eat at any of the fast-food chains. Here's how he recommends you get one.

Blame the manager, not the server. If you order fries but get attitude, "chances are strong there's something wrong with the management," suggests McNamara. "The manager is not respecting his employees. The mood of the manager often gets transferred to impressionable employees." If you get treated rudely, ask for the manager. Tell him or her what happened. Ask for either a replacement of cold food, your money back, or a gift certificate for free food in the future.

Call in a complaint—or a compliment. If you had bad service and want to complain, ask the manager for the number of the corporate headquarters. That should get their attention. The same goes for compliments.

Ask for a sound check. Curious that we can amplify the voice of the rock band Kiss to fill a 60,000-seat stadium but technology is unable to clearly transmit the voice of someone taking your order at the drive-up window? If you run into a communications breakdown at any drive-up restaurant, the best advice is to park the car, go inside, order your food in person, and give the manager an earful about what you couldn't hear.

you still are being ignored, walk up to the person who seated you and politely say you've been trying to get your waiter's attention for (fill in the blank) minutes or hours.

"Empathy always helps," adds Thompson. Such as, "Your staff must be swamped, but..."

Check on your check. Sometimes the longest wait is not for your food; it's for your check. "That's because the waiter may feel the hardest part of his job is over and he lets down," explains Weiss. Meanwhile, you have a life to get back to. He suggests telling the person who takes your reservation that getting the check promptly is of utmost importance, and reminding the host or maître d' upon arrival.

Betting on a Tip

The concept of tipping dates back to sixteenth-century England, according to John Schein's *The Art of Tipping*. You left coins in a container at pubs "to insure promptitude." Shortened to "tip," the idea caught on and spread to the United States by the late nineteenth century. Today it's a universally accepted custom—though it doesn't necessarily insure promptitude. But if you plan to go back to that same restaurant, you'd be well-advised to leave an appropriate gratuity. Or starve.

How much? That's usually the first question asked of Jerry Newfield, president of Tip Computers International, based in San Diego, which makes and markets a credit card–size plastic card that helps you tabulate tips (for more information, call 800-527-9493). Up until 1980, says Newfield, 10 percent was the appropriate tip. In the opulent early 1980s, it went up to 15 percent, then 15 to 20 percent by the mid-1980s. Now the rule of thumb is 15 percent for service, 20 percent for particularly good service, and more if you want a booth named in your honor.

How to Pass the Bar Exam

A man could go dry if he doesn't know how to get some respect when he sidles up to a bar. But if he understands the symbiotic relationship between himself and the man or woman serving drinks and good cheer, his cup will runneth over.

It's a two-way street, notes Lou Herborg, director of education at the Professional Bartenders School of New England in Boston, who has worked behind the bar at restaurants and country clubs.

"Respectful bartenders will never show you their backs," Herborg says. "They keep sweeping up and down the bar, making eye contact, keeping the energy up, making you seem like you're the most important person they're serving. They're your confidant, therapist, barber, big brother, father, and best friend rolled into one." Here are a few ways Herborg suggests that you can return respect.

Be inquisitive. Don't pretend you know what to order when you don't. "Good bartenders like to be of service," says Herborg. "That's why we do it." Ask for advice. Ask what's in a drink. Ask which are the better brands. To get you started, here's a primer on scotches. Bar, well, or house brands (such as Bankers Club or Lauder's) are the ones you get when you ask for "whatever you got." They're the least expensive and are usually on the bottom shelf behind the bar or under the bar. Call brands (such as Dewars) are of next-higher quality and on the next-higher shelf, followed by premium brands (Chivas Regal, for example) and super premiums (single malts such as Glenlivet).

Here are some additional tips on tipping.

Tip after, not before. That's the advice of Jean-Charles Benyahia, dining room captain at the Rainbow Room, high above Rockefeller Center in Manhattan. His reasoning: "Tipping

Buy your buddy a drink, not the bartender. "The last thing you want is a drunk bartender," says Herborg. If he accepted yours—and every other "buddy's" at the bar—that martini could start to taste like mud. So don't offer a drink to the barkeep (especially instead of a tip). It's actually considered a sign of disrespect. And, adds Herborg, it shows the bartender no disrespect if you turn down a free drink from him.

Mind your manners. If you want service, forget about the following: whistling, tapping a coin on the bar, yelling "Yo," or shaking your empty bottle or glass at him.

Drink at a leisurely pace. Don't order more than one drink at a time. That impresses nobody. And it's a waste of a good drink; by the time you get to the second glass, the ice will have diluted the drink. "We don't mind if you nurse a drink," says Herborg. "It shows you respect a good drink."

Go nonalcoholic. If you don't want alcohol—for any reason—you will win points (not lose them) by abstaining. Resisting even strong peer pressure earns big points. Whether you order a Perrier, virgin Bloody Mary, juice mixtures, or any of the finer nonalcoholic beers (such as Haake-Beck by Dribeck Importers or Kaliber from Guinness), you can still be a man among men and pass the bar exam.

Leave the driving to someone else. Respect your limits. If you do happen to go beyond the limits of sobriety, quietly ask the bartender to call you a cab. Or if you drove, ask a friend to drive you home in your car and pay for his cab back to the drinking establishment so he can get back to his car.

You leave a generous tip for extra special attention—only to find out all tips are pooled and your tip will be divided among the whole staff, no matter how lazy the others are. Not fair, you protest. Next time, you take the waiter aside and say, "This is just for you." If they're a professional, they'll say thanks—and still place the money in the pool. Benyahia offers this compensation: "Your generosity will be discussed, and next time you come in, even the ones who didn't wait on you will pay you the respect you deserve."

Stiff bad service, but tell the manager. When the service is so bad that the waiter does not deserve a tip, a mouse will stiff the staff and dash for the door. A man will not leave a tip and speak directly to the manager to explain why—in detail. Says Asimov, "Watch what happens the next time you go to that restaurant. The manager will practically serve you herself."

Give yourself some credit. Even if your waiter laughs hysterically and points to the fountain when you ask for a refill of water, you might still be subliminally muscled into giving him a fat tip. In a small study conducted in two restaurants, social psychologist Michael McCall, Ph.D., of Ithaca College in New York, found that people cough up more cash when the bill comes on a tip tray with a credit card logo—even if they're not using a credit card. "The insignia appears to convey the idea of credit or money," theorizes Dr. McCall. "People may come to associate credit cards with spending."

So how can you avoid this sneaky manipulation? Take a few seconds to shake off the gold-card hex, consider the service you've received, and then give as good as you got.

before feels like you're trying to buy me. I want to please you and feel like I've earned your respect—and your tip."

Dive into the pool. Here's the scenario. You've had the best waiter in years.

In a Store

Buying Into the Retail Scene

What is the smartest thing to bring into a retail store when you go shopping?

1. Your checkbook
2. Your credit card
3. Your lawyer

At one time or another, all of the above may come in handy. But the single most important item you can bring with you is knowledge of the product you intend to buy.

"The more informed you are *before* you make a purchase, the less you'll need organizations like ours *after* you make a purchase," cautions Stephen Brobeck, executive director of the Consumer Federation of America, a nonprofit consumer advocacy group in Washington, D.C.

When salespeople know that *you* know something about the product you're thinking of buying, not only will they have more respect for you but there will also be less of a chance that they'll pull a fast one on you.

Get in the Game

Do your homework. Research the products. Study the marketplace. Shop—but don't necessarily buy. Ask lots of questions. Scan newspaper ads. Page through trade publications. Surf the Internet where many companies now have Web sites. And don't forget good old-fashioned word-of-mouth recommendations.

Of course, getting you to put out all this energy may be a hard sell, considering shopping is not an activity men generally respect. About one in three men strongly dislikes shopping, according to a survey conducted for *Daily News Record*, the

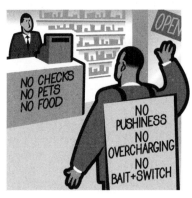

leading menswear trade publication. Another 24 percent are negative, but not to the same degree. Only 11 percent of men actually like to shop.

Our advice: Think of shopping as a sports event. From the moment you walk into a store, it's a one-on-one contest. There's some fast-talking salesman trying to lead a fast break to your hard-earned cash. You're looking for a steal. While he's dribbling away, you cut in, grab the ball (or in this case, a real nice 12-volt, pistol-grip, variable-speed drill with a keyless chuck, adjustable clutch, and infinite torque), dart toward the check-out counter, and slam-dunk a terrific buy. Score! Suddenly the entire sales staff holds you in the highest regard. Here are some scouting reports to help you get past that pesky salesman.

Fend off an aggressive salesperson. "Saying 'I'm just looking' leaves a hole for a pushy salesperson looking for a commission," warns David Cook, Ed.D., director of training and development for Sears Tire Group, a division of Sears, Roebuck and Company. He suggests putting it this way: "I'm here to just browse. If I need you, I'll look for you specifically. Tell me your name." That way, he points out, you've put them on notice that you know why they're being so pushy and that if you do want to buy, they'll get theirs, too. If they persist, either walk out, pride and disposable income intact, or go to the manager and politely report that that salesperson is ruining your shopping experience.

Beware the bait-and-switch. The ad said sale. When you got there, the product you wanted had just sold out. Oldest trick in the book. Or you tell the salesperson you have X dollars to spend and he keeps recommending the item for X-plus dollars. "When you get the sense that what you're saying is going in one ear and out the other, you can bet the bait-and-switch maneuver is on," Dr. Cook says. Hold your ground. Don't bite the bait. Respect yourself—and your financial limits.

Dress the part. If you want to get respect, don't walk into a store unshaven and wearing funky jeans. "Would you respect a salesperson who looked that way?" asks Dr. Cook. "Respect goes both ways." On the other hand, he warns, don't wear your salary on your hand-tailored sleeves. "If you look like you're worth a million bucks, that's how much they may think they can get you to spend," he adds.

Check it out. *Consumer Reports*, the magazine that rates products brand by brand, is a great source of information if you want to get the respect of the salesperson with whom you're dealing. "Without a question, it is the best independent source on consumer goods," Brobeck says. "It's well-funded, has the highest standards, and sells no advertising."

What's in Store for You

There are unwritten laws that govern the retailer's world. Unwritten, that is, until now.

"Men are like fish out of water in a store," says James Adams, the design principal for Seattle-based NBBJ Retail Concepts, a division of one of the country's largest architecture firms. "It can be a frustrating and intimidating experience." Knowing your way around a store will help you feel less like a stranger in a strange land.

Shop midweek. Wednesday is the slowest shopping day of the week, according to research Adams's company has conducted. So if you want lots of personalized attention, shop then. Saturdays and Sundays, not surprisingly, are the busiest shopping days. Though sometimes you'll see a bunch of salespeople on the floor on weekends, often one is the manager or assistant, two are full-time sales staff, and the other half-dozen are part-time help who may not be as well-informed as any of the two

---

Buyer Beware

Sometimes we earn respect by knowing what to do if and when a sale turns sour.

"Knowing the reliability of the store you're dealing with should be as much a part of your research as knowing what product you want to buy," says Holly Cherico, director of public relations and communications for the Council of Better Business Bureaus (BBBs) in Arlington, Virginia, the umbrella for the 137 BBB offices nationwide. Though the regional BBB offices cannot bring legal action, they can provide reliability reports that disclose how long the business has been in practice, how long the bureau has known about it, and whether complaints have been filed against it. The bureau also can offer assistance on how to resolve complaints. Cherico offers these suggestions.

- Make sure you understand the warranty and contract terms.
- Ask about refunds, return policies, and exchanges *before* you make the purchase.
- Keep all sales receipts and instructions.
- If a problem develops, speak up immediately. Don't call three months later about a product that was faulty when you bought it.

---

or three people you'll encounter midweek.

Get out of line. Here's a tip guaranteed to slash your shopping time: You can pay for an item at any open cash register. So always look for the shortest line.

Eyes right. What's the quickest way to find the men's section when you walk into almost any department or clothing store? Look right. "For some reason, people naturally will move to their right when they come into a store." Adams says. So that's where they put the menswear department to make it shopper-friendly for men.

At the Garage

Greasing the Wheels of Respect

Ever seen the motherboard of a computer? Tons of wires, delicate metal stuff, and funny looking chips. Well, your car has a kazillion motherboards. One works the brakes, another the fuel system, yet another the cruise control, you name it.

Not only do all of those wires, connections, and funny-looking chips make it nearly impossible for even the most mechanically inclined guy to fix his own car but they also give your auto mechanic a lot of power—power that can put the average guy in an uncomfortable bargaining position. To repair cars, a mechanic has as much automobile knowledge as there are words in 250 phone books. If he tells you your starter needs to be replaced because it is draining too many amps from your battery, who are you to argue? You have no way of knowing whether he's telling the truth or just making an excuse to install an expensive part in your car.

The best you can do is get the mechanic on your side. When a mechanic respects you, he'll do anything to keep your business. He'll explain your options more fully. He'll make sure your car doesn't get stuck on the lift for weeks. And he'll never pull a fast one.

Steering Clear of Trouble

Obviously, knowing as much as you can about cars helps, says Larry Webster, a self-proclaimed car nut since childhood and technical editor for *Car and Driver*. You can gain some knowledge by reading your owner's manual

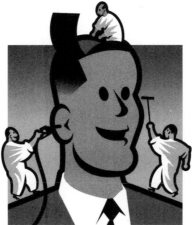

as well as books about cars, he says. But even if you don't know a rotor from a wheel cylinder, you can still forge respect. Here's how.

Poke around. When you go to a garage for the first time, let the mechanic watch you as you take a look at the certificates hanging on the wall. Look for ones that show that the garage and its mechanics are accredited by the American Automobile Association (AAA) and the National Institute for Automotive Service Excellence (ASE). Check out the dates on educational certificates. If the dates are recent, it means he is staying on top of the industry.

Then ask to walk through the garage. Look over his equipment. Ask about his recent purchases. If the guy hasn't bought any tools since he installed his lift 20 years ago, chances are he's going to have a tough time fixing your car in a timely manner, says Lisa Mayer, who owns Rick's Automotive Tire and Repair in Ballston Spa, New York, with her husband, Rick.

Question everything. Ask "why" often. For instance, if the mechanic tells you that your brake pads and rotors need to be replaced, ask "why?" It may sound like a stupid question, but it's possible that your mechanic can save you some money by turning your rotors rather than replacing them. If you don't ask why, you'll never find out your options.

If you have one of those ominous "he thinks I'm an idiot" gut feelings, pester him some more, Webster says. For instance, you can say, "I'm not knowledgeable about this, but for me to feel comfortable having you work on the car, I need you to take some time and explain exactly why I need a new transmission to pass state inspection."

Start with an oil change. The worst time to try to find a mechanic is when your car is broken. Instead, get to know him by taking the car in for small maintenance, such as oil changes and tire rotations, says Ron Ciglar,

A Guy's Guide to Car Problems

Want to sound somewhat knowledgeable the next time you head to Joe's garage? Think about what's actually wrong with your car. Then match your symptom up with the probable diagnosis listed below. With the guidance of Tony Lee, owner of Lee's Auto Service in Washington, DC, we've listed some of the common things that can go wrong, along with what causes them. Just remember: When you march into the garage, be careful not to tell the mechanics how to do their jobs. They hate that.

Symptom: You hear an unusual noise only when the car is running but not in motion.
Diagnosis: Engine problem.

Symptom: You hear an unusual noise only when the car is in motion, especially when going over bumps.
Diagnosis: There's something wrong either with your suspension (the car's support system that allows the wheels to move) or drivetrain (everything that holds the transmission and axles together).

Symptom: You hear a squealing sound when you start the car.
Diagnosis: A belt is slipping and either needs to be adjusted or replaced.

Symptom: You hear "click, click, click" whenever you make a hard turn.
Diagnosis: It's your constant velocity, or CV, joints, which are a part of the axle that moves the wheel.

Symptom: You hear a high squealing sound coming from the car when it is in motion.
Diagnosis: You need new front or rear brake pads.

Symptom: You try to accelerate when going uphill but the engine revs up without accelerating.
Diagnosis: If your car is manual, you may need a new clutch, and if it is automatic, you may need transmission service.

Symptom: You notice your headlights dimming or your windshield wipers slowing as you drive.
Diagnosis: Your alternator (the car's electrical powerhouse) is calling it quits.

Symptom: You try to start the car. You hear "click, click, click." The car won't start.
Diagnosis: Your battery is dead.

Symptom: You try to start the car. It won't start. You hear one loud "click."
Diagnosis: Your starter is broken.

owner of Ron's Automotive in Philadelphia, which was rated one of the most reputable garages in the country by National Public Radio's *Car Talk* Web site. When something major does happen to your car, a mechanic who knows your name and face will try harder to get your car fixed quickly than he will with some other guy with a blown head gasket who walks in off the street and wants it done yesterday.

Wash your car. Mechanics will often sum you up just by giving your car a once-over. If you routinely bring in a dirty, dented car that hasn't had the oil changed in years, your mechanic not only won't respect you but he'll also assume that you don't give a damn about how well your car runs, says Tony Lee, owner of Lee's Auto Service, which also is on the *Car Talk* list of reputable garages.

Prepare for manual combat. When you go to the dealership or the quick lube for regular maintenance, a technician will probably ask to change a whole mess of car fluids. Sure, changing your transmission fluid every day may make your car run longer, but not long enough to make it worth the money or time.

So show up armed with owner's manual in hand. And when the mechanic suggests some form of maintenance, check to see what your manual recommends and stick to it, says Webster.

Leave the diagnosis to the mechanic. Often, we tell the mechanic what we want done on the car, falsely believing that such an attitude will make the mechanic think that we're on the ball. But it usually makes the repair more expensive. "Eight out of 10 times, the customer is wrong when diagnosing their own car," Ciglar says. "The guy will say, 'I need new plugs. That's what the problem is. Put new plugs in.' We try to tell him that we don't think the plugs are causing his problem. But he won't listen. So we put the plugs in—even though the car doesn't need them—and it still doesn't run well."

Instead of trying to diagnose the car, me-

chanics would rather we provide symptoms. Provide a what, where, and when. For instance, if there's a funny noise, say where it sounds like it's coming from, what it sounds like, and when it usually happens, Lee advises.

Tell the whole story. You may not want to admit that you drove over a few parking abutments to see how well your new four-wheel-drive worked. Keeping such information from your mechanic, however, will only cost you more money and embarrassment. The guy is going to figure out what you did fairly soon after he gets the car on the lift or pops the hood. Plus, leaving out such information means that the mechanic must play detective. It will take him more time to diagnose the problem, costing you more money in the long run, says Mayer.

Get what you pay for. Because cars are so complicated, it's reasonable that a mechanic won't fix every problem the first time. So if something goes wrong after you get your car back from the garage, don't automatically storm in yelling obscenities. Just take the car back, explain that the problem is persisting, and wait to hear his answer. A reputable mechanic will take the car back and fix it free of charge. Or he'll refund your money for his initial work and only charge you for the repairs that were true fixes. If he doesn't offer such an option, ask for one. "I won't charge anyone unless what I do fixes their car," Ciglar says.

Play show and tell. Have the mechanic actually show you what he's talking about. If he's replacing a part, ask to see the old part and the new one side by side. Ask him to show you the difference between the two. And keep the old part (or if it's something huge like an engine, ask the mechanic to hold on to it) until you are sure the new part is doing the job. If a mechanic puts a new part in a car and it still doesn't work, then ask to have the old one reinstalled at no cost, Ciglar says.

Play favorites. Every mechanic has a group of favorite customers, customers for whom he would do anything to make sure that they never take their cars elsewhere for repairs. What's the easiest way to become a favorite?

Make the effort to establish more than just a business relationship. Ciglar loves the one guy who sweeps his garage while waiting for his car. He also speaks fondly of the woman who brings him cookies every Christmas Eve. Even the people who take time to make small talk become people he especially wants to keep happy.

Haggle with care. Sure, the mechanic can give some price breaks. For instance, some shops offer a 10 percent discount on the parts they stock. Also, garages calculate labor costs based on a guide that tells them how long various repairs should take. So if the guide says a brake job should take a couple of hours and the mechanic gets it done in 1, he has the choice of charging you for the 2 hours or only charging you for the time it really took, Mayer says. But keep in mind that the mechanic is the one laying down the cash for tools and equipment, and he isn't getting a break from anyone. Mechanics will be more likely to cut you a break as a way to thank you for your patronage if you're a regular customer whom they can respect.

The thing is that mechanics won't respect you much if you keep badgering them about price. Second only to chronic check-bouncers, a mechanic's least favorite customer is the guy who thinks car repairs are as negotiable as car purchases. They're not.

When all else fails, get a second opinion. If you know that something is wrong with your still-under-warranty car and the dealership keeps giving the thing a clean bill of health, or if some mechanic is recommending a

huge price tag for repairs that just don't sit well in your brain, have another garage look it over, says Webster. One option is a diagnostic center operated by the American Automobile Association. They will inspect your car and try to find the problem. Because the center doesn't do repairs, you know the mechanic there won't suggest a ton of replaced parts unless your car really needs them.

Avoiding Unnecessary Work

Nothing will gain a mechanic's respect quicker than knowing what maintenance work is necessary for your car and what isn't. Here are three common repair-shop services that your car—and your wallet—can live without, says Jeff Shumway, master mechanic and author of *The Answer: Getting More and Paying Less for Auto Service*.

Forget the 3,000-mile oil change. Unless the $19.95 oil change special includes a car wash *and* a free ice scraper, don't bother. Most cars will do just fine if you wait until the manufacturer's specified interval in the owner's manual (usually every 7,500 miles).

Stop rotating your tires. "People think it makes their tires last longer, but it doesn't," says Shumway. "If your tires are wearing unevenly, rotating them won't fix the problem." One caveat: Some tire manufacturers will void your warranty if you *don't* rotate your tires at specified intervals. Check your warranty.

Don't fall for the "drain-and-fill" routine. This is where they drain the old coolant (usually half antifreeze and half water) from your car's radiator and replace it with 100 percent antifreeze, which can eventually cause engine damage. Instead, have your existing coolant tested. If it fails, ask them to replace the original mix.

On an Airplane

How to Be Treated like a Jet-Setter

Some carriers have gone the extra mile to try to win passengers' respect by attempting to improve the quality of notoriously bland food and making seats more comfortable. The proof, of course, is in how much respect *you* feel they're giving you—not in the slick advertising or puffy press releases. As Ed Perkins, editor of the *Consumer Reports Travel Letter,* says, "A lot of people are sold on the sizzle rather than the steak."

There are steps you can take to make your next flight smoother, from reservation to destination. Here's what the experts recommend.

Making Reservations

Don't peak. That is, call at off-peak hours if you want to avoid the purgatory of being put on hold. That means before 8:00 A.M. or after 6:00 P.M., Midwest Express spokesperson Lisa Bailey says. To be safer, call even earlier or later. And don't get impatient if you are put on hold. If you hang up and redial, you'll move to the back of the line. Be forewarned: When you're making reservations to travel during peak travel times—major holidays, the height of vacation season—it's every man for himself. The worst times are one or two days before and after the holidays. But the actual day of the holiday (Christmas Day, Thanksgiving Day) is strangely quiet. If you can, book to travel then, and you'll have the plane practically to yourself.

Save a seat. Booking a seat when you book your

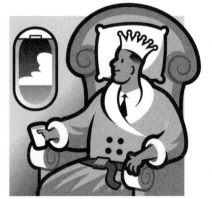

flight is a good idea, Perkins says. If you can't afford a first-class seat, you can hold out for the better of the coach seats. For extra room, Perkins suggests the rows right behind the emergency exits on most wide-bodied and a few narrow-bodied planes. The bulkhead rows right behind the cabin dividers are another good option, and they offer a bonus: You won't have the person in front of you breaking your kneecaps when he reclines his seat.

Take names—and numbers. If it's not offered, make sure you ask for your locator number. Also get the full name of the person who is making your reservation, and if you're really skeptical, request the name of that person's supervisor or manager. At the end of the transaction, make sure the information is repeated—and write it all down. This is your insurance policy in case you call the next day and a new reservations agent says that the conversation you had the day before was a figment of your imagination.

At the Airport

You arrive at the airport, adrenaline pumping. Point A (curbside) looks a long way from Point B (your seat). Here's how to navigate through the obstacle course known as the terminal and still maintain your dignity.

Travel light. The savvy traveler can pack a week's worth of wardrobe into a carry-on bag, leaving room for at least one more carry-on, such as a laptop, briefcase, or gym bag. Each airline has its own rules about the number of carry-ons allowed and their sizes. Check when you reserve your flight. This way you avoid waiting in line to check your bags—and repeating the frustrating drill on arrival at the baggage claim area. It also eliminates the opportunity for the airline to send your luggage to a nicer locale than the one to which you're heading.

Bypass the ticket

counter. If you have checked your luggage at the curb (or only have carry-ons), already have your ticket (or have booked through electronic booking), and had the foresight to reserve a seat when you booked, go directly to the gate, check in there, and wait for the rest of those fools back in the terminal to catch up to you.

Join the club. Most airlines have so-called private membership clubs. For about $200, you can join. That entitles you to hang out between, before, or after flights at the carrier's lounge in the airport. "One delay or layover and you'll feel that it's money well-spent," says Randy Petersen, editor of *InsideFlyer*, the magazine for frequent fliers. Most clubs have workstations with phones and computer hook-ups, comfortable chairs, and complimentary hot drinks and soft beverages.

On the Plane

You've heard us say it before: To get respect, you must give it. But perhaps nowhere is that truer than at 20,000 feet. "When we sense that people respect how hard our jobs are, we bend over backward to make their experience with us more pleasurable," says Sharon Wingler, a flight attendant since 1970 and author of *Travel Alone and Love It*. Here are some ways to earn respect a mile high.

Watch the show. What is the number one pet peeve of flight attendants? According to Martha Minter, director of in-flight services training for Alaska Airlines, it is that "nobody ever watches the safety demonstration." Take 30 seconds, watch the flight attendant run through the drill, make eye contact, smile, let her know you're watching, commiserate with the fact that no one else is paying attention, and throw in a "thank you" as she walks by.

Up with Upgrades

Upgrades are the way to make sure that you get respect on flights. But contrary to popular mythology about how to get that treasured first- or business-class seat, "groveling is out, networking is in," says Randy Petersen, editor of *InsideFlyer*. Here's how to work your way toward the front of the plane.

• **Take advantage of service problems.** The next time a flight is late or delayed, the food is cold, or the staff is not friendly at all, think about what you want. "The right answer is not a $25 fare certificate, not 500 bonus miles," advises Petersen. "The correct answer is an upgrade for later on. Why? These are often good against any fare code, and also you can confirm them at the time of booking."

• **Call or eat your way to an upgrade.** Sign up to earn miles from your telephone service or from one of the many restaurant programs sponsored by the airlines. With the miles that come from these types of partners, you can get confirmed upgrades without harm to your normal miles earned from flying, Petersen says.

• **Change partners.** Some hotel and car rental programs give their best customers complimentary membership in an airline partner's elite-level program. Elites often get gratis upgrades of the standby type (depending on the program) and access to other types of upgrades.

• **Take what you're entitled to.** One of the biggest trends in airlines is to give free upgrades based on the fare you pay. "If you are a last-minute kind of flier and pay big bucks for that coach seat, shop around for the airline that gives confirmed upgrades for full-fare coach ticket purchases," Petersen suggests.

Remember the magic words. "It's so simple to earn respect," says Wingler. "Make eye contact and be polite. You'd be amazed at how far 'please' and 'thank you' and a little courteousness will get you."

Ask—it couldn't hurt. You want the whole can of tomato juice or ginger ale? Ask for it politely. You want more peanuts? Ask graciously.

Around the World

How to Avoid a Culture Clash

The story is told today that the folks at Coca-Cola had a little bit of trouble when they decided to bring their world-famous beverage to China in the 1920s. Instead of choosing characters in the Chinese language that would describe the flavor of the drink, it seems execs originally tried to use ones that sounded like the English name. In a master stroke of obfuscation, those Chinese letters ended up translating as "bite the wax tadpole" or "wax flattened mare."

Needless to say, something got lost in the translation. When it comes to relating to other cultures, such dilemmas are all too common—and perhaps never as common as when you're talking about respect.

You see, fellow travelers, if there's one thing that people around the world don't quite understand or appreciate, it's our relaxed American manner. To them, backslapping is crude and verboten. "They assume that when you're that friendly, it implies a lot of commitment, mutual trust, and responsibility—that it's a lasting and ongoing relationship," says Hilka Klinkenberg, author of *At Ease...Professionally* and managing director of Etiquette International, a Manhattan-based corporate consulting firm.

Tips for Travelers

Here's how to command respect when you're abroad—and possibly avoid an international incident.

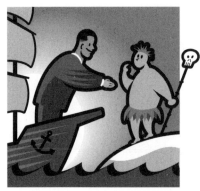

Put the sir in surname. It sounds extremely formal, but before greeting anyone by their first name, it's best to ask permission. "Calling someone by their first name in most other cultures is totally unacceptable," Klinkenberg says. "It's considered a real invasion of privacy." It's better to err on the side of caution and use the person's last name (their surname) unless they tell you otherwise. Canadians and Aussies don't really mind, but really watch yourself in Scandinavian countries. Using someone's first name without their permission there is almost as bad as dying your hair black and refusing to eat cheese.

Give Klaus and Mario proper credit. When calling on a German client, make sure you know all of his titles—and use them—lest you risk a show of disrespect. "If he has a Ph.D. and is the director of a company, you would call him the equivalent of Mr. Dr. Director and his surname," says Klinkenberg. Italians prefer to be addressed by both their profession and their surname.

Be an "exchange" student. Americans pass out business cards like they're trinkets at a Mardi Gras parade. Not the Japanese. Their great respect for corporate culture has turned exchanging business cards into a procedure not unlike an economic summit. As a result, before greeting a business client in Tokyo for the first time, it's a good idea to have your business cards translated into Japanese.

When presenting your card, hand it with two hands with the printing facing him. Do not, repeat, do not, simply grab his card and stuff it into your wallet or back pocket. Instead, study the card for a few moments and resist all temptation to write on the back—that's also considered an insult by the Japanese. When you've given it sufficient consideration, place it carefully in your top shirt pocket.

What happens if you

somehow blow the Great Business Card Exchange? You may not be toast in Tokyo business, but "they are going to look at you rather warily. They are on their guard at that point because you have been somewhat insulting. You have treated them as if they are inconsequential...their business card is a serious representation of who they are," Klinkenberg says.

Avoid eye contact. Another routine American practice makes the Japanese uncomfortable: staring into their eyes. "They perceive that as staring them down, trying to intimidate them," Klinkenberg says. Chances are that your Japanese host will fix his gaze somewhere between your chin and the tip of your nose. You should direct your gaze to the same area on your host's face.

Get the signal. Frustration over language barriers often causes us to use hand gestures to try to get a point across. But you can get in all kinds of trouble around the globe if you indiscriminately flash the handy "okay" sign. Wave one in France, and they'll think you or something else is a zero. If you try it in Japan, make sure that your other hand is on your wallet: There it means "Time to talk money." Worst is Brazil, where it refers to a certain part of a woman's anatomy unmentionable in a family-friendly book series. "It's considered very vulgar and obviously should be avoided," Klinkenberg says.

Be a space cadet. Invading someone's personal space can be a big no-no in some cultures. "As a general guideline, the farther north you are, the more distance there is between people when communicating," says Marjorie Brody, a certified speaking professional, co-author of the *Prentice Hall Complete Business Etiquette Handbook,* and president of Brody Communications, a business and communications skills training company in Elkins Park, Pennsylvania. "Among those who typically stand closer than Americans are people in the Middle East, Latin America, Italy, Russia, France, and Spain." (It might be a good idea to keep the breath mints

handy the next time you're in Saudi Arabia— for yourself, if not your host. Arabs may stand as close to you as two to three inches. "If you back away from them, it's an insult," Brody says.)

Save your sterling. You may lose your shirt in a game of darts the next time you're in an English pub, but at least you don't have to tip the bartender. "If you do, you'll get strange looks and they'll know for sure you're a tourist," Brody says.

Save your sole. If your travels take you to Thailand, don't show anyone the bottom of your feet. "They're the lowest part of your anatomy, and the signal is that whoever you are pointing them at is beneath contempt. That goes for all Arabic cultures as well," says Klinkenberg. So what are you supposed to do if you find yourself sitting on the floor? Try tucking your feet under so you're sitting on your feet and your knees. "A friend of mine was in Pakistan sitting for hours on the floor of her friend's house. When she got sore and had to stretch her legs, they would get all flustered and throw a rug over her legs. And she would say, 'No, I'm hot.' But they would do it anyway because she was showing them the soles of her feet. And they were only doing that because they were friends. Otherwise, they would have been extremely offended."

Shake, don't break. Your massive forearms may give you the Handshake of Doom, but leave it at home when traveling abroad. The French and Germans only want one quick pump from their handshakes, and then it's over. "Anything else isn't considered a lack of respect, but you're perceived as being gauche," Klinkenberg says. And don't be surprised if your Japanese guest hands you a day-old squid. "When someone here gives you one of those limp fish–type handshakes, we assume they are untrustworthy, dishonest, lacking confidence, and all sorts of things. But that doesn't apply to the Japanese. They are not a touch culture. They have made the accommodation to our style of greeting," says Klinkenberg.

At a Party

Merry-Making Made Easy

A long-overdue moment of silence, if you will, for the ultimate party animal, Bluto Blutarski.

There.

And while we're laying dear Bluto to rest once and for all, it's probably a good idea for us to leave his *National Lampoon's Animal House* party habits behind as well.

Now don't get us wrong: We enjoy draining a brew and crushing it on our forehead with one hand as much as the next guy. And taking a whiz outside in the bushes? Forget about it.

But we're grown men now—many with families, jobs, revolving forms of credit, and malfunctioning garage door openers. If we're truly going to command respect at a party, we can no longer behave like beer-swilling frat boys. At least not until the wife and kids go to her sister's for vacation.

The Life of the Party

To help guide us gently into this respectable party environment, we've turned to Mary Mitchell, author of *The Complete Idiot's Guide to Etiquette* as well as the "Ms. Demeanor" column syndicated to newspapers throughout the United States; Hilka Klinkenberg, managing director of Etiquette International; and Barbara Pachter, president of Pachter and Associates in Cherry Hill, New Jersey, and co-author of the *Prentice Hall Complete Business Etiquette Handbook*.

Be clothes-minded. Since clothes help make the well-respected man, you have

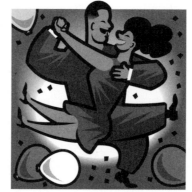

to wear the right threads for the occasion. By now, even the fashion victims among us should know that an invitation that says "formal" means it's time to break out the tux—or hit the rental counter. To some, "black tie optional" may sound like an opportunity to forgo the monkey suit, but to others it's an opportunity to shine.

"What usually happens is that the host or hostess would like to say black tie, but they're afraid they're going to alienate guys who don't have a tuxedo or don't like to wear them," Klinkenberg says. "But if you come dressed in a tuxedo, you're just going to look more polished and savvy." Semiformal or informal, according to Klinkenberg, has you decked in a white shirt with French cuffs, cuff links, and a subdued dark tie and suit. Most cocktail parties require informal dress. Casual could mean everything from a sport jacket and khakis to flip-flops and dungarees, but when in doubt about the dress code for any party or get-together, ask your host or hostess beforehand.

Go easy on the sauce. Sure, it's a party and the idea is to have fun. But nothing costs you points on the respect-meter quicker than liquor. "I don't care what anyone says, two drinks should be your maximum," Klinkenberg says. "I've been told by people that they can drink anybody under the table, but they're also getting more and more boisterous. You may not fall over flat, but staggering doesn't look profes-sional, savvy, classy, or respectable." Your lack of control also puts added pressure on your host, who now has to worry about how you're going to get home and whether you're going to get in a fight with an impor-tant client he has spent the last six months wooing.

Avoid hors d'oeuvre overload. At a swank cocktail party in a New York City museum, Klinkenberg recalls watching aghast as people piled so many hors d'oeuvres on their plates that the food was falling off. "This is unprofessional conduct, folks," she says. Her helpful hint: One layer of hors d'oeuvres per plate is enough. "You don't have to take it all the first time—they let you go back for more. But the buffet or bar, for that matter, should not be the first port of call or the main focus of your attention at a party," she says.

Stuff the stogies. Cigars may have staged a comeback in many trendy restaurants and bars, but you won't find them on the guest list at most parties. Light up, and you're likely to see your respect level go up in smoke. "You shouldn't be smoking those things at a party unless the host is," Klinkenberg says. "It's disgusting...and proves you're a boor, that you don't know how to behave in polite company."

Keep your distance. Now that you know that a guy who commands respect isn't afraid to hit the dance floor (if you missed that part, see Self-Respect on page 38), we expect to see you make an occasional appearance. Just remember to treat your dance partner with respect— especially if you've just met. "You don't have to crush someone against you to lead them around the dance floor," Klinkenberg says. "It makes a lot of women very uncomfortable when some fellow pulls them that close. This isn't a bump and grind session."

Keep your jacket on. The temptation is to peel off that jacket, roll up your sleeves, and get down to some serious partying. But not if you want to command respect among those in the know. "Only after dinner, and only if the host does. If your host isn't taking his jacket off, you're not supposed to," Klinkenberg says.

Don't hijack the host. When you first arrive, a natural tendency is to spend a lot of

---

Give Yourself a Hand

How many times has this happened to you?

You're confidently waxing philosophic on instant replay in the NFL, with a drink in one hand and a plate in the other, when Mr. Important approaches.

Eager to shake, you quickly juggle your libation, only to grip him with the coldest, clammiest hand in history and drop onion dip on his suede shoes. He recoils in horror, speechless. You apologize profusely—but later that same evening discover that you've been removed from the lucrative Oldmoney account and replaced by a summer intern.

We feel your pain. Now you, too, can partake of food and drink—with napkin to spare—while maintaining a warm, dry hand perfect for shaking. Simply follow this technique, suggested by Hilka Klinkenberg, managing director of Etiquette International.

- First, place your napkin between your ring and baby finger of your left hand.
- Now, spread your middle finger and ring finger, placing your hors d'oeuvre plate between them. Allow your index finger and thumb to rest on top of the plate.
- Place your glass between your index finger and thumb.

Ta-da! You're now a one-handed party animal. "Everything is in your left hand, and you take it into your right hand as you need it," Klinkenberg says. "That way when you are introduced to somebody, you are smooth and in control. It just works wonderfully well."

---

time hobnobbing with the host. Bad move. "You should try to talk to him only briefly, but once he introduces you to other people, you know it's time to talk to other people," Klinkenberg says. "Part of the reason he's introducing you to someone else is so he can make his escape and do the rest of his hosting duties."

Sing for your supper. Some guys go to a party expecting to be entertained. The fact is, a good guest is supposed to help bring the party to life. "You're supposed to socialize and mingle, to talk and basically be upbeat. And that means that you introduce yourself even if no one is talking to you," Klinkenberg says. "If you're at a social party, you can talk a little longer, but if you are at a business party, you should really keep it to 5 to 10 minutes because part of the point of the exercise is to network and mingle."

Be a weather guy. Unless you're fast on your feet, the party could be over before you dream up the ultimate conversation starter. But you can't go wrong if you open with something safe and simple, like the weather. "You can find out a lot about a person with a topic as seemingly banal as the weather," Mitchell says. If you offer that you're not fond of the heat because you're from Antarctica, it's legit to ask how summer's treating them and where they're from. And once you have that down, you can ask how they ended up living here.

Do your best Larry King. Simply asking lots of follow-up questions is the best way to keep the conversation going. Throw in a "really?" or "wow" or "tell me more" every half-minute or so—rather than launching into your own monologue—and you'll be the life of the get-together. "I call these words 'prompters' because they prompt people to talk," Klinkenberg says. Other tricks you can use include asking open-ended questions that require a sentence to answer, such as: "So, what's your favorite episode of *Xena: Warrior Princess?*" Avoid a questioning tone of voice or critical sentence structure as in "So, what do you mean you don't like Xena the Warrior Princess?"

Exit, stage right. Lest you think we've lost our sense of humor, note that we've obviously seen *Animal House* more than once, own a prized boxed set of Three Stooges episodes, keep abreast of the latest political wisecracks, and know our way around more than a few Top Ten Lists. But when it comes to racist, sexist, or demeaning jokes, we're outta there. In the event someone starts to tell one in your presence at a party and you're not interested, Mitchell says you can make a quick exit by saying, "I don't want to hear this" and moving away. If you don't realize what kind of joke it is until it's too late, look at him squarely without laughing and respond with, "I don't think that was the least bit funny." It may cause some controversy, but at least you acted with integrity.

Make a preemptive strike. It's great to reminisce, but there's nothing more boring than a pointless, poorly told war story that you've already heard. So the next time Commander Farnsworth tries to regale you with tales from his Albanian campaign, you have to act fast. Respectfully—but fast. "Try something like, 'Oh, this is that great story about how you were captured behind enemy lines. That must have been quite an experience,'" says Mitchell. "Then jump in with a new topic of conversation."

End well. "When you feel a conversation has run its course or it's necessary for you to move along, wait for a break in the conversation, then say, 'Well, I have to say hello to our host (or George or my aunt, for example),'" says Mitchell. "Or say, 'That food looks delicious. Think I'll have some' or 'I'm going to the bar for a refill.' (Don't try this one while holding a full glass.)"

Put it in writing. The food was exquisite, the conversation engaging, the tribute to beach volleyball queen Gabriella Reece first-rate. Comforting words, all—yet they're only likely to garner maximum respect and appreciation if you put them in writing on a note card and send it the day after. (With a gift of flowers, perhaps?)

"If you want to look terrific, if you want to stand apart from the crowd, always, always, send a hand-written thank-you note," says Pachter. "It only needs to be a few lines: 'Thanks for the great party. I really enjoyed the food and the company.' Pretty basic, pretty simple, but it makes such an impression."

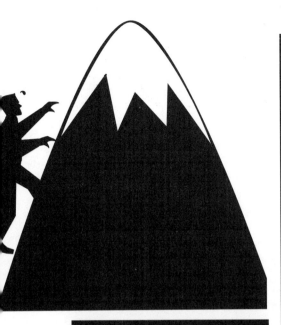

Part Six

Real-Life Scenarios

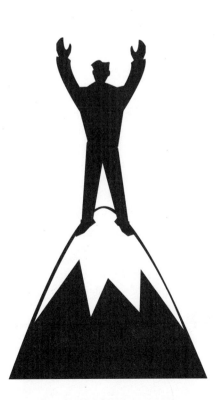

Quest for the Best

These men are more than just celebrated and successful. They are respected. Against the odds, they have climbed to the top of their professions without compromising their integrity. Here are their stories.

You Can Do It!

If declining respect is the problem, these guys—and the thousands more like them across the country—are the answer. Each day, they command respect by quietly working to make the world a better place. So can you.

Quest for the Best
These men are more than just celebrated and successful. They are respected. Against the odds, they have climbed to the top of their professions without compromising their integrity. Here are their stories.

Rabbi Harold Kushner, Bestselling Author

A Good Man Shares His Wisdom

Can you respect a man—a man of the cloth, no less—who dares to question whether God deserves our respect? Yes, when that man is Rabbi Harold Kushner.

"When I pray to God, it's not because I think He has the capacity to heal me or you only if I find the right words to grovel sufficiently," Rabbi Kushner says. "I could not respect a God like that. I could not respect a God who could save an innocent child but refuses to because I didn't grovel enough. I would have nothing to do with a God like that."

A slight, soft-spoken man with glasses and thinning gray hair, he does not present the appearance of someone up to taking on God. Or even, for that matter, of becoming a highly respected public figure. But there he was, for example, representing the Jewish faith at the National Prayer Service in Washington, D.C., marking President Clinton's second inauguration. And there he is on the lecture circuit, speaking to business groups and at universities.

Rabbi Kushner rose to prominence in the early 1980s for speaking on behalf of any and all good people who feel they have been given a bum deal, the short end of the stick, a streak of bad luck. His book

When Bad Things Happen to Good People was written, he tells us in its introduction, "by someone who believes in God and in the goodness of the world...who was compelled by a personal tragedy to rethink everything he had been taught about God and God's ways."

In the simplest of terms, stripped of theological mumbo jumbo, Rabbi Kushner wrestles with trying to make sense of the death of his son, Aaron, at age 14 of a rare disease, progeria, which drastically accelerates the aging process. Finding particular solace in the book of Job, he concludes that the appropriate response to why bad things happen to good people is "to forgive the world for not being perfect, to forgive God for not making a better world, to reach out to the people around us, and to go on living despite it all."

The People's Rabbi

"I'm affirming God's goodness by compromising God's power because I think goodness is an admirable trait, not power," he

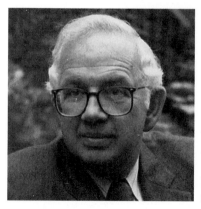

now says. "Power doesn't impress me. It can intimidate me. But I don't want to worship power. I don't want to aspire to power. I would rather aspire to goodness."

The book obviously struck a chord. It sold more than a million copies in hardcover and was published in 12 languages. Members of the Book-of-the-Month Club listed it as one of the 10 most influential books of recent years. Since then he has also written *When All You Ever Wanted Isn't Enough* and *How Good Do We Have to Be?*, among others. In recent years, he left as spiritual leader of a congregation in Natick, Massachusetts, to devote all his time to lecturing and writing.

The Natick temple's loss is everyone else's gain. "A vocational inventory I took early in college said that I should be an accountant, but I always knew that I was meant to do something more significant, more prominent than that," he says, adding in his introspective way, "Do we ever understand the life decisions we make?" He attributes his desire to become a rabbi directly to his rabbi, a man he respected and admired, and as a way to show respect to his own religious father (without having to go into his father's business).

It's the ease with which he admits to grappling with the fundamentals of life that so many others take for granted that has earned him such high respect—even by those who would be the last to declare themselves spiritual pilgrims.

"I could never write about human frailty and sinfulness if I hadn't experienced it myself," he confesses. "People often ask me if being religious helps you cope with misfortune, or do the rich have it easier than the poor, or the young easier than the old? It's none of the above.

"The key is self-respect," he goes on. "If you think that you're basically a good person, when something bad happens to you, you just brush yourself off and say, 'Well, that was a bit of bad luck, but hopefully tomorrow will be better.' If you lack self-esteem, your response is, 'I knew it. I deserve it. These things always happen to me. I'm never going to make anything of myself.'"

So the question, then, is how do you gain self-respect?

"My sense is that other people are the mirror in which we see ourselves reflected," Rabbi Kushner says. "So find yourself a community in which you are liked. You probably did it in self-defense in high school. There's

something almost instinctive about it. Find groups of friends who give you feedback that you're okay because the rest of the world isn't likely to do that. It's something that happens in the 12-step programs—finding people who will accept you with all your flaws. The cliché is 'I'm not okay, you're not okay, but that's okay.'"

Getting Real

It was only when he and his wife, Suzette, were thrust into the role of bereaved parents that he discovered the emptiness of many of the clichés he was using to try to soothe the grief and suffering of others. "I was saying things as a rabbi and I thought I was helping people, and I was shocked and dismayed to be on the receiving end and find out how unhelpful all those clichés are," he recalls.

"Now I show more respect by talking less and hugging more," he says. "I listen really well. I remind myself that every single person who sits across from me or who I see in an audience is fashioned in the image of God. They may be cranky. They may be exasperating, sick, and smelly, but they are mirrors of God and I can't let myself forget that."

And when you're the one in need of support, having a community that affirms your own sense of worth can help keep your tragedy from turning into what Rabbi Kushner calls "a life-debilitating experience."

The death of his son has also given him a greater respect for life. "Our mortality makes every day of our lives significant because we know that we have time in limited quantities," he says. "Every decision is an important choice, knowing that choosing one thing may mean not having the other."

Almost as a symbol of his life-affirming message, Rabbi Kushner dedicates *How Good Do We Have to Be?* to his grandson, born to his daughter in 1993.

As they say in Hebrew, *l'chaim.* To life.

Carlos Santana, Guitarist

Respecting the Note

The note. There is nothing Carlos Santana respects more than the note. He learned that as a young boy growing up in Tijuana, Mexico, whether playing violin in his father's mariachi band in grungy clubs on a Saturday night or in a church group the next morning during communion.

"The circumstances may have been vastly different, but the intention was the same: to pay the highest respect to the note," says one of music's most noteworthy guitarists, sitting in his management and production offices in San Rafael, about 15 miles north of San Francisco.

In sports it's called The Zone. In acting it's called The Method. In spirituality it's called Oneness. Respect for the note isn't just playing in tune and on the beat. It even goes beyond playing with richness, tonality, vibrato, and other musical terms. It's about playing the note with such depth and feeling and concentration that it becomes an almost-transcendent out-of-body experience. And hearing it—well, let the maestro explain.

"Certain musicians know how to respect the note so that when you hear it your heart surrenders," Santana continues, his big brown eyes wide with sincerity, his curly dark hair escaping from his familiar multicolored skullcap. He rattles off a bunch of exemplary names from whom he learned, a veritable who's who of legendary musicians: Nat "King" Cole, John Lee Hooker, B. B. King, Miles Davis, Bob Marley, John Coltrane. "You can't just play over the note. You have to be inside the note. Then people's hair stands up. They cry, they laugh, and they dance at the same time. They're healed, released from whatever

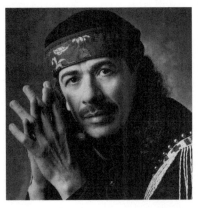

negative stuff they're carrying."

That's what respecting the note is about, he says, "an affirmation of your intentions, your feelings, emotions, and passion. Miles, Coltrane, and Bob Marley all taught me to shoot with my music for something beyond good and evil. To shoot for the fourth dimension, where you see that it's all in harmony and perfection."

True to His Beliefs

"I respect him because through all his evolutions, he has remained true to himself and his beliefs," says Ben Fong-Torres, the San Francisco journalist who was music editor of *Rolling Stone* magazine from the late 1960s to the early 1980s. He interviewed Santana several times during those heady days of the San Francisco rock scene. "His core character is a highly spiritual person who feels strongly that through music and one's behavior a higher purpose can be filled."

On top of all that, "he was the first major figure from San Francisco's Latino Mission District to succeed commercially. Creatively, he expanded rock's vocabulary the way B. B. King and Paul Butterfield and Otis Redding did. He imbued Latin influences into rock in a seamless style," adds Fong-Torres, author of an autobiography, *The Rice Room: Growing Up Chinese-American—From Number Two Son to Rock 'n' Roll.*

Santana has proven that he was no flash in San Francisco's Panhandle, headquarters of the Grateful Dead, Janis Joplin, and Jefferson Airplane, among others. Since 1969—with his introduction to the world on the stage of Woodstock and the release of *Santana* (4 million sold) and *Santana: Abraxas* (*Playboy*'s jazz and pop record of the year)—he has won nine gold albums as well as a handful of platinum disks. While he treasures his various music-related awards, Santana is even more proud of such citations as the Outstanding Leadership Award from the National Hispanic Heritage Week in 1986 and a 1991 resolution from the California State Latino Legislative Caucus honoring his "outstanding contribution to the arts and his true commitment to the Latino community."

At the forefront of the benefit rock concert trend since 1972, he has performed for free to raise money for such causes as Nicaraguan earthquake victims, Live Aid, Amnesty International, the children of El Salvador, and many more. He and his wife, Deborah, are foster parents to a dozen young people around the world. To honor the town where it all started for him, he still supports a skills training program in Tijuana for troubled children.

Respect Begins at Home

It was from his father, Jose Santana, that he first learned to respect the note. Though his father recorded only once, with Carlos on an album called *Havana Moon*, "they called him Don Jose, a term of respect, in his community," recalls Santana. "I admired his dedication to music as well as to our family. He made me practice the violin every day. I hated the violin. But out of respect for him, I played."

A day of emancipation came while he was playing in one of those smelly clubs with his father in Tijuana. "These were the worst places you could imagine. I felt like vomiting. I've never told anybody this before, but I can't stand certain Tex-Mex music because it reminds me of those days. So I told my father I didn't want to be there or play this music anymore. He could have done one of two things: break the violin over my head or suck it up and let me go. To his credit, he let me go."

But it was his mother, he says, who had the vision. "Everything I am I owe to my mom," he says. She was the one who got the family out of the tiny Mexican town of Autlan, then out of Tijuana to settle in the San Francisco area in 1962. "From my mom I learned that if you can see it, you can paint it; if you can hear it,

you can play it," he explains. "She saw a bigger stage for us."

It was his mother who pulled him across a plaza one day when they were still back in Tijuana to hear something new. A guitarist was mimicking the twangy sound popularized by Duane Eddy and other American musicians. "It was like seeing a flying saucer or having a close encounter," he recalls. "I said, 'This is it. This is who I am for the rest of my life.' That was the beginning, a door."

He opened the next door when he arrived in San Francisco. Washing dishes by day at a restaurant, playing nights and weekends at weddings, bar mitzvahs, and in vacant alleys, he went one night to hear blues guitarist B. B. King perform at rock impresario Bill Graham's new Fillmore in San Francisco. "The guy got a standing ovation before he even played a single note," Santana says. "And then he played. For me it was a revelation: the blues the way it was supposed to be played—from the heart!"

While many consider Santana a Latin-inspired musician who successfully fused Latin, rock, blues, and jazz sounds, he prefers to pay his respects to the continent from which almost all rhythm-based music descends: Africa. "If you draw a map and trace any music—Jamaican, Brazilian, Spanish, Indian—all the lines are going to start from Africa," he explains. "Call it salsa or flamenco or reggae or jazz or blues—it's all African music."

And what does he call his music? "I call it gumbo," he smiles. "But hey—guess what? It's all one. That's my music's purpose. To make people wake up, take a deep breath, and digest and accept this: We're all part of the same totality. We're all brothers and sisters. So why would the Protestants want to fight the Catholics, the Palestinians fight the Jews, the White man fight the Black?"

At the televised *Billboard* awards ceremony in December 1996, Santana characteristically used the national exposure to spread his message. "Treat each other with dignity, harmony, compassion, and love," he suggested. "That is the key to the new millennium."

John S. Hendricks, Cable Television Magnate

His Discovery Leads to Respect

He's been called the conscience of cable television, his channel "the most respected name on TV," according to a poll of viewers. But more than anything, John S. Hendricks, founder, president, and chief executive officer of Discovery Communications, has shown that, despite what the sharks in TV-land say, programs suitable for you and your kids can garner high ratings and financial success.

In fact, from the early days of renting and broadcasting well-made but dusty documentaries, Hendricks has grown his company into a worldwide media empire—with channels or programs in more than 140 countries. In addition to the Discovery Channel, the company operates The Learning Channel and the all-nature Animal Planet and Discovery Channel International. Then there are the ancillary products, such as Discovery's retail chain, the Nature Company; Your Choice TV, an on-demand viewing service; and Discovery Online, the channel's award-winning Web site. The sum revenue of all these and other Discovery ventures in 1996 topped $600 million.

Yet no one seems as amazed with his success as the former Huntsville, Alabama, resident. "I'm much more intimidated today. I know all the reasons why it shouldn't have worked," Hendricks says.

In the Beginning

To gain the same level of appreciation, flashback to the late 1970s. Hendricks was just a 20-year-old work study student putting in his time in the University of Alabama's history

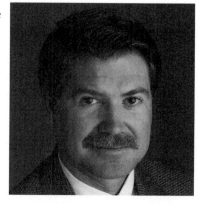

department when he discovered the idea for Discovery.

"One of my jobs was to get 16-millimeter films for some of the faculty to use in the classroom," he says. "So I became familiar with all these film catalogs from the BBC and Time-Life films and all these wonderful documentaries that were in the catalogs." Much to Hendricks's dismay, too few of the documentaries in those catalogs ever appeared on television.

A few years passed, but Hendricks never lost his fondness for those films. And when Time successfully challenged the law preventing cable providers from broadcasting their own content in a bid to create HBO, Hendricks astutely recognized that the television landscape was about to change. And that he might want to be a part of it.

"Around 1980, I read that Ted Turner was going to start a news network and someone else was going to start a sports network.... It was in April 1982 when I just thought, 'When is someone going to start a documentary channel?'" he says.

Hendricks began researching the ratings for documentary programming on broadcast and public television. He liked what he saw. The folks who watched educational programming were better educated and wealthier than the typical TV viewer—a fact he figured advertisers were bound to appreciate. Even though he wasn't sure what to call his concept—he chose the name Cable Educational Service to incorporate in 1983—Hendricks was certain that he was on to something big.

The venture capitalists Hendricks visited to ask for money for his cable channel were skeptical. And they pointed to CBS's cancellation of *Universe*, a documentary-style program hosted by television anchor/icon Walter Cronkite, as a good reason not to invest.

After hearing this same argument over and over again,

Hendricks tried to get actual ratings for *Universe*. When that effort failed, he decided to ask the icon himself—Cronkite. Instead, he reached Cronkite's secretary, who sympathetically urged him to write a letter and spell out his intentions. She assured Hendricks that she would make sure Cronkite read it.

Hendricks wrote the letter, and a few days later, the phone rang. "I pick it up and it's Walter Cronkite," Hendricks recalls, still slightly in awe. "He thought a documentary channel would be terrific, and he was telling me all the reasons he thought it would work. And they were the same reasons I thought it would work."

Armed with his research, a letter from Cronkite endorsing the idea, and a new name for the service—"It was between Vista, Horizon, and Discovery"—Hendricks signed up enough investors to make the channel happen.

Just as it appeared that his dream would become reality, a major investor suddenly pulled out, leaving Hendricks unable to pay his small staff. But Tele-Communications Incorporated (TCI), one of the largest cable providers in the country, and two other cable companies, Cox Communications and Advance/Newhouse, came to the rescue, providing the cash needed to position the fledgling channel for growth.

Playing with the Big Boys

No media magnate's story is without controversy, and Hendricks's tale is no exception. In a suit that was eventually dismissed, the creditors of a defunct channel called The Learning Channel accused Discovery and TCI of "anti-competitive use of monopoly power." It seems that after Lifetime signed a letter of intent to purchase The Learning Channel for $39 million, TCI wouldn't guarantee that its cable outlets would continue to carry The Learning Channel.

When the deal with Lifetime fell through, Discovery eventually bought The Learning Channel for $32 million—a price that Hendricks

still maintains was fair. But at least one media analyst says the deal gained the attention, if not the grudging respect, of the industry. "It was clear to observers that the amiable Hendricks was now playing in the rough, tough big leagues," wrote Warren Berger in an article in the *Los Angeles Times*.

If art imitates life, a closer look at Hendricks's very private life reveals a man committed to learning and helping to bring out the best in his employees—as he all the while maintains a firm grip on the reins of power. His day often starts at 8:30 A.M., mulling the contents of four leading newspapers. He's also a voracious reader of nonfiction, recently working on a biography of Lewis and Clark of expedition fame.

He'll often greet employees who work in Discovery's Bethesda, Maryland, headquarters by name—even though there are 700 workers at that location. And he's rarely seen flying off the handle, managing instead with what Discovery's vice-president for communications Jim Boyle describes as "calm confidence." But he has been known to get peeved when someone tries to grab credit at the expense of others. "That kind of grandstanding bothers him," Boyle says.

And he's not shy about pushing an idea of his own. Known around the company for sketching designs for products, Hendricks personally designed the logo that now graces the Discovery Channel.

A typical night of Discovery programming—from "Lions, Tigers, and Bears, Oh My!" to "Seeking Jesse James" and "Hyenas: Nature's Gangsters"—sounds more like what your mom or your fourth-grade science teacher would want you to watch than standard TV fare. But that's the idea.

"We've been able to build a business by creating what we think is an informative, quality product. We knew it wouldn't be for everybody, but in a way almost everybody at some point during the week is in the mood to learn," Hendricks says. "And when they are, we're ready."

Mic Rodgers, Stuntman

Laying It on the Line

For a decade, he has been *the* stunt double for Mel Gibson and the second unit director/stunt coordinator all the studios call when they need serious movie magic. In his biggest challenge to date as a second unit director, he personally managed the painfully realistic battle scenes that helped win *Braveheart* an Academy Award. And if all goes as planned, he'll be the man directing a few of the blockbusters coming soon to a theater near you.

But to hear Mic Rodgers talk, none of that is quite as important as what his father told him before he died of cancer. And what has been reinforced time and again on television and movie sets from Hollywood and Miami to London and Israel: Be there for your brothers in the business, Mic. And be willing to give it all back.

"I am a high school graduate, the son of a truck driver," says Rodgers. "And I stumbled into this almost by accident. Now I've done my part to get where I'm at on the physical and mental level, but a lot of guys have taken the time to help me out. They said, 'You have potential. I'm going to help you.' And now that's what I'm trying to do."

Breaking In

Growing up in the Los Angeles suburb of San Gabriel, Rodgers never even thought about working in Hollywood. But because he was dyslexic, anytime his teachers allowed the class to work on a student play or film instead of turning in an English paper, Rodgers was game—especially since a friend's father made it so convenient. "His dad had a camera shop, and every time a 16-millimeter camera came in, he would hold it for an extra week

so we could use it," Rodgers recalls.

When the teens tried to perform more daring stunts for their films, it occurred to Rodgers to ask a pro how it was really done. And that led him to his first mentor in the business, Paul Stader. "He ran sort of a stunt school, but it was more like you became part of his entourage, one of his protégés," Rodgers says.

Soon after, Stader brought Rodgers to the set of the blockbuster disaster film *The Towering Inferno*. "Paul was the stunt coordinator for the show. One minute I'm just standing around watching what's going on, and the next minute I have a fire extinguisher in my hand. Then Steve McQueen, one of my heroes, walks by and I'm like, 'I can't believe this!'"

Although Rodgers already had a full-time job as a mechanic's helper at a tractor dealership, he slowly took on more stunt work. "I came in at a good time," says Rodgers. "There were tons of TV action series on...*The Dukes of Hazzard, Wonder Woman, Baa Baa Black Sheep*. So someone my age, 23 or 24, could be a guard, or a soldier if that's what they needed. I'd cut my hair. It didn't matter."

Before long, Rodgers found himself running from Universal and Warner Brothers to Twentieth Century-Fox, performing stunts five days a week. But it wasn't just the thrill of steady work at something he loved that made it great. "Every day we were learning something new. How to coordinate stunts—without any prep time or money. So when I broke into features, it was easy. They give you so much time and so much money and you think, 'Wow, I could have done this with $1.95 and a roll of masking tape.'"

Since his first two years in the business, Rodgers has never worked fewer than 300 days a year. And it shows. His seven-page résumé, meticulously kept up-to-date by his wife Robyn, includes appearances in everything from *Baywatch* and *The Bionic Woman* to *Matt Houston* and

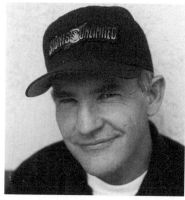

*M*A*S*H*—as well as dozens of others shows, mini-series, and made-for-TV movies. And—oh yeah—more than 150 feature films.

Learning His Craft

If it was Stader who got Rodgers into the business and taught the 6-foot, 185-pounder how to get flattened without breaking too many bones, it was a director named Richard Donner who became like a father to him. Not only did Donner hire Rodgers for stunts on the first *Lethal Weapon* movie but the veteran producer also seemed to be grooming him for even bigger things.

On the set of films such as *Scrooged, Lethal Weapon 2, Lethal Weapon 3*, and *Maverick*, Donner mentored his younger, soft-spoken friend. "I'd stand around the set and watch them shoot dialogue scenes. And he'd say, 'What would you do with these actors?' And I'd say, 'I would do this or that.' Then he'd say, 'Go tell them. It's a good idea.' He was semi-training me to express myself, to speak up about things that I thought weren't my domain. It was good stuff."

Rodgers's training continued in earnest after Mel Gibson tapped him to be second unit director on *Braveheart*. His first responsibility on the film: whipping 1,500 regulars from Ireland's version of the national guard into shape for the climactic battle scene.

After two weeks of training—just moments before Gibson was to arrive to inspect the troops—Rodgers gave a pep talk that sounds like it would have done Patton proud.

"I went to one side and told them Mel was coming to see the test battle, and they were the Scots. And those guys on the other end of the field were the English. And so they were booing them and making all kinds of noise. And then we walked down to the other side, and I said, 'Okay, you guys down here, *you* are the Scots and those guys over there are the English.' They were all freakin' out."

When the two celluloid armies clashed, Gibson's mouth fell open. "It was unreal," says Rodgers. "It took 3 minutes to stop them. And everyone was screaming and using bullhorns going, 'Cut, cut, cut.' And they were still going at it. Broke every sword we had."

While Rodgers's movie life is certainly full of action and glamour, those things pale in comparison to the friendships, trust, and respect that he has developed for his fellow stunt performers over the years. "When you're asked to join Stunts Unlimited (a fraternal stunt organization), you take the oath to be a brother to the other members. Now you may have a personality problem along the way with some other member, but you have to put that aside and hire him if he is the right guy for the job," Rodgers says.

And that brotherhood extends to both good times and bad. Members who are hurt or disabled often have their bills paid or are given money by the other members. In one such situation, a stunt performer who developed cancer and couldn't work for a year had his mortgage paid by the group.

Such generosity is hard to imagine—until you remember that stuntmen and stuntwomen routinely risk their lives for one another. "Respect to us is if I say I'm going to be somewhere at a certain time, I'm there. Or if you say, 'I have to light myself on fire for this scene,' I'll promise you that I will put you out before you get burned, no matter what. I'll do that. I'll sacrifice my body or my life to keep a guy from getting hurt. That's what commands respect."

And in the same way that Stader and Donner and Gibson mentored Rodgers, he's giving back now to a young man named Chris Tuck. "When Chris got out of high school, he came out here to live with my wife and me," says Rodgers. "He's 25 now and on the verge of becoming a great stunt guy. He doubled for Bill Paxton in *Twister*—did all the car driving. In 10 years, he might find someone to pass it on to. Who knows? He might pass it along to my son, Cooper. You have to pass it on. You have to replace yourself. If you don't, it's like bad mojo."

Millard Fuller, Habitat for Humanity Founder

Building a Better World

A self-made millionaire by age 29, Millard Fuller had it all. "2,000 acres of land, horses, cattle, speedboats, a Lincoln Continental, a maid.... It was a very plush lifestyle," he recalls.

Until a personal crisis led him to give it all away. "Business to me was exhilarating and exciting, but I was in such a headlong pursuit of wealth that I was totally out of balance," he says. "It's like an alcoholic can't taper off; you have to leave it alone. And I just had to leave it alone."

Fuller abandoned his financial quest, but he didn't leave success behind. He founded a nonprofit organization called Habitat for Humanity, an empire of dreams built on donations and the sweat of volunteers and would-be homeowners. Exemplifying what Fuller calls the Theology of the Hammer, Habitat has built or renovated more than 50,000 homes, making it the nation's fourth-largest home-builder.

Giving It All Away

Habitat's official goal is impressive: "To eliminate poverty housing and homelessness from the face of the earth." It is, to say the least, an ambitious goal. Some would even call it quixotic. "At Habitat we say there is a difference between faith and foolishness. But we encourage people to get as close to foolishness as possible without crossing the line," he says. "We're a long way away, but what we're beginning to do is eliminate poverty housing and homelessness from certain places. It is starting to happen."

Born "in the small cotton-

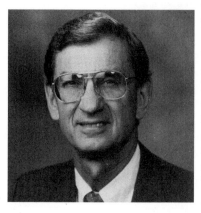

mill town of Lanett, Alabama," Fuller was raised with Christian values, regularly attending church on Sunday. When he arrived at the University of Alabama, Fuller says, "Like a lot of college students, I left Jesus at home and got very interested in making money." Lots of money. He and a friend found a mind-boggling variety of ways to pursue their financial aspirations—from running an on-campus birthday cake delivery service to renting, buying, and building student apartments. In 1964, at the age of 29, the married law school graduate had reached what many even today would view as the pinnacle of success: He was worth more than a million dollars.

But as the money poured in, his personal life disintegrated. Fuller's wife moved out and threatened him with divorce. Not only that, his health was faltering. He suffered neck and back pain, kidney problems, and shortness of breath. Sometimes he had to grab the arms of his chair and focus on filling his lungs with air before he could relax and breathe normally.

Fuller sensed he needed to take action. He had his company pilot rent a plane and fly him to New York City. There, he met with his wife. They saw a show at Radio City Music Hall and, afterward, through many tears, agreed to reconcile. But that was just the beginning. During the taxicab ride to the hotel, Fuller proposed giving the money away. All of it. Without hesitation, his wife agreed. "We felt God was calling us to divest ourselves of our wealth and go seeking His path for us."

The couple took a two-week vacation together driving down to Florida. Along the way, Fuller decided to visit a Christian community in Americus, Georgia. It was there that they met the community's founder, Clarence Jordan, author of a series of translations of the New Testament called *The Cotton Patch Versions*. The visit turned into a two-month-long stay—and a friendship was formed that would alter the course of Fuller's life.

Taking Jesus Seriously

Following a three-month trip to Africa, where he and his wife toured mission projects, Fuller continued redistributing his wealth. The cash went to a host of projects, including short-wave radios for mission stations; a dorm and library at a small black college in Mississippi; helping resettle displaced Uganda Indians; and a fund to send young short-term missionaries to other countries. "It was so meaningful for me and my wife to go and see that work; we wanted to make it possible for other young couples to go and then come back and be spokesmen for the work," he says.

Jordan had some work planned of his own. He wanted Fuller to return to help turn 42 acres of Koinoia Farm into a development of not-for-profit houses for poor rural families who were being displaced by agribusiness. Money for the houses would come from donations and no-interest loans from benefactors. The farmers would slowly pay the money back as they were able. It was a radical idea, but Jordan had more than a few of those.

"He took Jesus seriously," says Fuller. "He reminded us that Jesus never said the first and great commandment was to go to church. He said the first and great commandment was to love God with all your heart and mind and soul and strength and your neighbor as yourself. So it was a new understanding of my faith." That understanding led Jordan and Fuller to begin what was then called partnership housing. Before the first house was completed, tragedy struck: Jordan died of a heart attack. But his teaching was etched on the heart of his friend. "I had my eyes opened at Koinoia Farm to the fact that a full-bodied Gospel of Jesus had to be more than singing and talking about it," Fuller says.

Hammer Time

After a three-year term of missionary service in Africa, Fuller founded Habitat for Humanity in 1976—probably the only organization of its kind to ever receive help from the likes of everyone from Jimmy Carter and Bill Clinton to Newt Gingrich and Jack Kemp.

New Habitat for Humanity affiliates—local groups organized to build homes for needy families—are being added at the rate of 10 to 15 a month. Family selection committees review applications from people who are homeless or live in substandard housing and who are unable to obtain conventional financing. As funding and land become available, families are chosen to receive Habitat houses.

Volunteers working with the chosen families build simple, decent homes of solid, quality construction. True to the model set at Koinia Farm, the houses are then sold without profit or interest. But the family that receives a house must perform what's called "sweat equity"—they must work several hundred hours to help build their own houses and the houses of others.

Government funds are not accepted for the building of the houses, "to ensure the grass roots strength of the work and so that the ability to function as a Christian program is not compromised," he says. Government help is solicited and gladly received for such items as land, streets, sidewalks, and for some personal and administrative expenses.

"You can hear how people who have lived in squalor, with overgrown yards, amid junk cars and unrelenting hopelessness, vow not to let a piece of trash on their property, and you experience the dawn of human dignity as it is born within them," says Fuller. "While people differ on theology and philosophy and politics, we can agree on a hammer as a way to bring us together. That's the Theology of the Hammer. Everyone needs a simple, decent place to live.... The boldness of the goal stirs people, and each year we are amazed at what fresh miracles come from such boldness."

Fess Parker, Actor and Entrepreneur

Blazing New Trails on the Frontier of Respect

In the small pantheon honoring mythical male heroes, right there next to Superman and Rocky Balboa, stands Davy Crockett. When they inducted him into the Mythical Male Heroes Hall of Fame (also mythical), we assume you were there, wearing your furry coonskin cap, improbable raccoon tail dangling from the back (come on, we know you've kept yours). And when the congregation started wailin', *"Dav-yyy...Daaaa-vy Crockett..."* we know you instinctively sang the next line without hesitation: *"King of the wild frontier."*

You could not have been alive in the 1950s and 1960s and *not* known of Davy Crockett. He was a certifiable icon, with America's playrooms full of Davy Crockett merchandise to prove it. He was a man who commanded our respect by virtue of his values, his integrity, and his ability to grin down a bear. Consider these nuggets of wisdom from the films *Davy Crockett, King of the Wild Frontier* (1955) and *Davy Crockett and the River Pirates* (1956).

- "Half of any battle is knowin' you're gonna win."
- "We gotta win this race fair and square."
- "He ain't never quit nothin' in all his life." (Spoken by his sidekick played by Buddy Epsen.)
- "You know me—when I'm sure I'm right, I go ahead."
- "Next time I get up before you, I'll have something to say worth sayin'." (Spoken by Crockett the first time he took the floor in Congress.)

The Myth and the Man

Based on the early nineteenth-century trapper from the backwoods of Tennessee—who went on to become a U.S. representative and then died heroically defending the Alamo in Texas—Crockett will forever be linked in modern times to Fess Parker, the lanky and laconic actor who starred in the early TV miniseries and the movies that followed.

In the plastic fantastic world of Hollywood, playing the part of a man of integrity is one thing. Playing that part in real life is quite another. But that's the role Fess Parker has played since immortalizing Crockett and, in a later TV series, another American folk hero, Daniel Boone. In the years since he stopped acting, he has become a highly successful businessman, buying real estate, developing hotels, and starting an award-winning winery. Along the way, he has amassed considerable wealth while earning admiration for achieving it all with typical humility and integrity.

Carving out a life after show business wasn't originally his idea. After working six years on the *Daniel Boone* TV series, Parker says, he was informed he would receive "no profits then, now, or later." This was not his understanding of the contract he had signed. "The creative bookkeeping you've heard a lot about in Hollywood was the order of the day," he now says. "They just threw me out and treated me only as well as they had to."

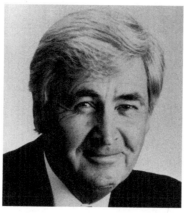

Seeing the Machiavellian handwriting on Hollywood's wall, convinced he was shut out, he was forced to consider other options. "I just thought it was time for me to be with my family and pursue new interests," he says. "And, over a period of time, I realized that adversity couldn't have given me a better opportunity."

In 1962, he started buying real estate. His first dealings

were in Santa Clara, California, 30 miles south of San Francisco. That turned out to be the heart of what became Silicon Valley, the West Coast epicenter of the computer industry. Not a bad investment. Later, he acquired land in Santa Barbara, on the scenic coast 90 miles north of Los Angeles, which later became the retreat of choice for many a Hollywood type. In 1986, he developed, designed, and opened Fess Parker's Red Lion Resort across the street from the beach in Santa Barbara. It's now called Fess Parker's Doubletree Resort.

Aging Like Fine Wine

In 1987, he juggled still another entrepreneurial ball, purchasing more than 700 acres of land in the Santa Ynez Valley, 40 miles north of Santa Barbara, and establishing the Fess Parker Winery and Vineyard in the little town of Los Olivos.

Though the winery's 1994 chardonnay, pinot noir, merlot, rieslings, and syrah wines have won a number of gold, silver, and bronze awards, Parker is most proud of watching his son Eli (Fess Parker III) emerge as one of the top wine-makers in the region.

"I've seen my son develop a talent, mature, and take leadership, and that was worth all the time and forbearance required to make a winery profitable," says Parker. Today Eli is president of the winery; Fess serves as vice-president of marketing, a responsibility that includes signing autographs for young and old Davy Crockett fans.

Married only once (he and his wife, Marcy, have been together since 1960), Parker also has a daughter, Ashley, a mother of two, who is active as a volunteer with the Ronald and Nancy Reagan Family Fund in Santa Barbara.

"Fortunately, this family is extremely blessed with good health and good prospects," says Parker, whose 6-foot-6 frame belies a gentle nature and a soft voice still laced with his native Texas twang. "I know that it doesn't get

any better than this in life."

It was on the Texas farms and ranches of his youth, where he was born in 1924, that Parker learned the ropes of respect. He absorbed a work ethic from his grandfather and father. Of his grandfather, he still recalls being impressed with how many people crammed the church at his funeral.

"I knew him as a loving man but never realized how much people looked to him in the community," says Parker. His father served as the local tax assessor and later as a county commissioner. His parents were also active in community affairs as members of a number of organizations "whose backbone was a moral standard and doing of good deeds in the community."

But what he got most from his family, he adds, "was the sense that I could go anywhere and accomplish anything I set out to do."

The word *respect* evokes from Parker a contemplative, "Hmmmm...interesting word.

"To me it means a man may not agree with you, but he'll be fair in his assessment of your point of view," he finally comments after a long pause. "It involves keeping promises."

Of his old Hollywood associations, Parker mentions two men he respects from his generation: James Garner and Clint Eastwood. "Both have done really good work. Garner has given us an awful lot of entertainment and some serious acting along with it. Clint has had a vision of his career and stuck to it."

As for the respect the public continues to shower on Parker's Crockett and Boone, "it all begins with the moral center of those characters."

That moral center, he goes on, was "essentially the Golden Rule": Do unto others as you would have them do unto you. "Those men knew how to solve disputes among men, between cultures and between relationships within the family and friends," he explains. "That was a constant of the series."

And you can bet your coonskin cap that those parameters will always be constant when future kings of the wild frontier define respect.

You Can Do It! If declining respect is the problem, these guys—and the thousands more like them across the country—are the answer. Each day, they command respect by quietly working to make the world a better place. So can you.

Building Back Respect

Brian Sasci, Fort Lewis, Washington

Date of birth: December 31, 1959

Profession: Army Warrant Officer maintenance technician

I've been in the Army since 1978. I've also been in the Boy Scouts much of my life—as a scout and now as a leader.

Parents and mentors are up against a lot today—insolent celebrities-run-amok conspire to strip respect from our society. Communities like the military and the scouts build it back.

Both the military and the Boy Scouts are organizations steeped in respect. Soldiers share a great respect for this country and for doing what's right. They're willing to give their lives for it.

Respect may be the backbone of the military, but not because we wear rank on our collars. When push comes to shove, all the stripes and stars in the world don't matter. Respect must be earned—one person at a time.

In the Army Now

I didn't come from a rich family, but my itchy feet yearned to travel overseas. When the Army called, I answered and enlisted right out of high school. I haven't been disappointed; I've traveled all over the United States and Europe. Also, I quickly realized that many of the things that I enjoyed in the Boy Scouts were waiting for me in the Army—the same sense of responsibility, the same call for order, the same devotion to respect.

Many times in the Army I have looked upon fellow soldiers with respect and felt a surge of pride knowing that I have earned theirs. One memory really stands out in my mind. In 1990, I was deployed with 20 soldiers to Laverno, Italy, to repair vehicles for a peace-keeping mission in Bosnia. We were sent on a seven-day mission—which stretched out to 90 days. The soldiers were outraged! They had only brought clothes for seven days. They had told their kids they'd be back next week. And they turned to me for answers.

I talked to them in small groups to solve the most immediate problems. "Hey, these are the cards we were dealt," I reasoned. "Let's get the job done and go home." I talked to groups who hung out together because I had different relationships with each group. I learned who needed more clothes, who needed time off to call family members back home, who just needed a break. That's how respect is sustained—through personal relationships. We worked through their immediate concerns, completed the job, and returned home in good spirits—just in time for Thanksgiving.

The challenge of the military is that as you rise in rank, you supervise more and more soldiers, growing increasingly distant from those that you lead. When a battalion commander, the silver leaf insignia of a lieutenant colonel gleaming on his hat in the sun, stands in front of his 600 troops and gives an order, they're going to listen. But they'll follow where he leads because of the times he went to their workplaces and earned their respect by watching what they were doing, listening to their concerns, and answering their questions.

Respect is earned through honesty in one-on-one relationships. I couldn't tell you a celebrity or politician I respect, not because I don't imagine they're good people, but because I don't really know them. On the contrary, I respect my father and my uncle because no matter how good or bad I was as a kid, they were up-front and honest with me. That's how I live my life. I treat soldiers, scouts, and my kids as I like to be treated—with honesty and respect—no games, no hiding, no secrets.

It's especially a challenge these days to teach kids about respect when sports stars vie for kids' attention by being the biggest, baddest guy on the block. It's difficult to tell kids that's wrong when these guys make more money in a season than I'll see in my entire life. But I've learned how, through honesty and trust.

Everything I Learned...

I learned much of this in the Boy Scouts. Honestly, I didn't want to join the scouts—when I was a kid it wasn't the cool thing to do. My dad wanted me to join the Boy Scouts. I was nine, so I did.

The Boy Scouts taught me how to get along with other people and the importance of flexibility. In a troop of over 100 kids, you learn to adapt quickly. Or you go home.

Now as a scout leader, I see the bigger picture. Scouting teaches boys to organize themselves into patrols, to treat others courteously, to be trustworthy. Most important, it molds them into good citizens.

I see a lot of good kids in scouting, and a lot of bad ones, too. Those actually are the ones who need it the most. Scouting gives parents a tool to teach their kids to take responsibility for their own actions. Since it's a boy-run program, the scouts are at the helm. Leaders like me are just there to keep them safe. We can point them in the right direction, but it's up to them to get the job done. If a boy forgets his sleeping bag, he's going to get cold. (Within safe limits, of course.) But he'll learn to be more responsible next time.

You can talk about responsibility and respect to kids until your face turns blue and their eyes glaze over, but really you have to show it

to them. Sometimes you have to be blunt. Once my niece got detention in school for tossing a pencil on her teacher's desk instead of politely handing it to her. My niece couldn't understand why the teacher got so upset. Later that night when she was doing her homework at the kitchen table, I dropped a pen right by her papers. Her anger flared. Just when she was about to snap, I calmly said, "That's exactly what you did to your teacher today. Do you see how that was disrespectful?" She understood.

In the military and in scouting, I've visited different places and met people of distinct cultures—I joined the military to travel and see the world, after all. I've served in Fort Drum, New York; Fort Riley, Kansas; and three assignments in Germany. Theirs is a very different army. Since the German army has been around for a much longer time than ours, there's a lot more history and tradition.

Along with their traditions, German soldiers are a lot more formal, and they have a much more set way of doing things. They address each other very properly, for example. In an extraordinary way, though, the formality makes the soldiers closer. I think it's because the boundaries between ranks are so much clearer. The soldiers in our Army push the boundaries every day. They love to test their leaders to the limit. They force us to earn their respect.

But earning it is so important. Respecting others, and knowing that we have their respect, allows us to live our lives more happily. It gives us faith that we can trust each other and know that we don't have to look behind us every second to make sure that no one is pointing a knife at our backs. We can trust people to do the right thing.

To trust people, and gain their trust, I treat everyone as individuals. I try to find one thing about every person I meet that I can relate to. When there's a common bond in the center of your relationship, you can work on the stuff around the edges.

After all, the more people that you can get along with, the more pleasure that you get out of life.

Stopping the Cycle of Violence

Azim Khamisa, La Jolla, California

Date of birth: February 10, 1949

Profession: International investment banker

Not many fathers follow in the footsteps of their children. On January 21, 1995, the path my life was on changed forever. That night, I lost my only son, Tariq.

Tariq was a college student who delivered pizzas on the weekends to earn extra money. A 14-year-old boy named Tony Hicks was with three gang members when they decided to rob my son. They demanded the pizza. When he refused, they shot him in the back.

He died instantly. I felt like a nuclear bomb had detonated inside of me when I found out. It brought my entire life to a screeching halt; my mind and body shut down like all energy had drained from my system. I was just totally paralyzed.

My grief was so overpowering; I had to just yield to it. An experience like this really takes you back to your core. I temporarily lost all faculty of thought. It was a tough day, to say the least.

Fortunately, I had been meditating throughout this ordeal, so after his body was placed in the chapel, I was able to talk to him and feel his presence. I knew that he was happy and in a good place—in a better place than we are. And so there was a little solace in my meditation.

I really wasn't able to process any of my emotions until the day after the funeral. I recall that one of the first feelings I had was anger. My rage was not directed at Tariq's assailants, but at society as a whole. When I finally recovered and was able to think, I wrote a very emotional letter addressed to society.

Soon thereafter, I learned more about Tony. He had been a victim of gang violence long before my son. Both of his parents had been involved with gangs, but things were looking up for him; he had been living with his grandfather, Ples Felix, a city project manager in San Diego, for the past five years. From day one, I saw two victims on the end of the gun that killed my son.

I realized that for me, an eye-for-an-eye type of revenge wasn't going to make me feel any better. I was never angry at the kids who killed my son. Instead, I was angry at society for having created an environment that lets these kids end up in gangs, hurting themselves and other people because they don't have any other options. Society failed both Tony Hicks and my son.

Revelation on the Mountain

As a father, I kept thinking about how I wasn't there to help my son on that fatal night. What could I do for him now? As an Ismaili Muslim, I believe that prolonged grief impedes the journey of the departed soul, so you're much better off doing a good deed in their memory because good deeds are like spiritual currency. They are transferred to the soul and help fuel its forward journey.

Before Tariq died, I was a successful investment banker, often working 100 hours a week. By May 1995, I had wound down my business and decided to spend five days alone in the mountains. I needed to think about how and why I would live the rest of my life because my life just seemed very impossible. There on the mountain, I was struck with an idea to start a foundation in my son's name that would work to raise community awareness about gangs. The Tariq Khamisa Foundation could help a lot of kids and create spiritual currency for Tariq's soul.

Kids learn from example, so I knew that they would study my actions if I was going to show them that the cycle of violence could be stopped. When you "walk your walk" and you "talk your talk" and you are teaching by example, it's effective. What is not effective is when you end up pointing a finger at these kids and are very condescending. That doesn't work. Then your message just goes in one ear and out the other.

I decided to meet with Tony Hicks's grandfather, Ples Felix, to tell him that I had no animosity toward his family and about my vision for the foundation and how it could combat youth violence. When I walked into the room, he quickly took my outstretched arm and said that my reaching out to him was like a prayer answered. He had been praying for me and my family every day. He offered his help in any way he could.

I invited Ples to come to my house and speak at the next meeting for the foundation. My whole family was in town for the event. That night, our meeting was the lead story on the 11:00 news; they began the story by showing the two grandfathers shaking hands, my dad and Ples.

Now Ples works with the foundation regularly, and I think one of the most important things the kids see is Ples and me working together. We have a special program about gangs that we take to the local schools. During the program, after I give my remarks and before he gives his, we hug each other. It's how we salute each other every time we meet. We don't shake hands, we hug each other. And the kids see that. I think they expect us to have a more typical response to one another, which would be an eye for an eye. And here they see me working with Ples, trying to save children. That gets their attention.

We also made a video that's part of the program. Tony Hicks is in it, delivering a very emotional speech at his sentencing where he begs for my forgiveness and God's forgiveness and warns other kids to avoid the path that his life has taken. He also talks about what his life is like now that he is serving a prison sentence of 25 years to life. After the video, I get up there and tell them, "I'm sorry on behalf of all us adults. I have to apologize to you because we really have not done a good job for you. But now, having said that, I also need to ask you to help me." And one of the things I ask them in

my speech is to help me break the cycle of violence. Every time I've asked that question, the student crowd has responded with a resounding "Yes."

Love and Respect

I firmly believe that 14-year-olds are not born gangsters. They have it in them to be heroes. But in our society, our youth have lost respect for themselves and one another. I think that 90 percent of love is respect.

Recently, on what would have been my son's 23rd birthday, we made a special presentation to the kids at Tony Hicks's old middle school. We had bought this big tree to plant there in memory of Tariq, along with another 100 potted plants for kids to plant in memory of the people they had lost to gang violence. All the plants went in 45 minutes. We had to go out and get some more. There was one girl there who had lost three sisters. Afterwards, the school told us that they had a week of peace like they've never had.

The restorative aspects from this outreach have been incredible. We receive so many letters, boxes full of letters from the kids who have seen our program. Every time we save one child from committing an act of violence, we save two lives. None of this would have started if my son had not tragically died. I always remember that every life we save gives meaning to his life.

I'm often asked about what our society needs to heal itself. In a nutshell, I believe we need to stand up to the corruption of our ideals. When you lose your ideals, for greed or power or money, people don't respect you. As a society, we need to be able to have heroes who can say, "I won't allow this to happen, at any cost; I'm not giving up my integrity."

That's what happened to my son. He stood up. He knew that it wasn't right for kids to rob him of a pizza without paying for it. He was brought up to know what is right and what is wrong. He didn't have any confusion there. I'm very proud of him.

Fanning the Flames of Respect

Ronald Richards, Forest City, Pennsylvania

Date of birth: September 11, 1956

Profession: Assistant to the superintendent at the State Correctional Institution at Waymart, Pennsylvania, and state fire instructor and volunteer chief of the Forest City Fire Department

I became interested in the fire service when I was a kid. My father was a member of a local fire department, although he rarely fought fires. His role was more administrative. Where I lived, there wasn't much for a kid like me to do. So I joined the fire department the first chance I got. You had to be 16 years old to join. I couldn't wait for my 16th birthday when I could submit my application. I had seen a lot of people who were in the fire department for a year or two and then dropped out for one reason or another. But it was more than just a passing interest for me. I wanted to make a career out of it.

To me, a firefighter is someone who is willing to take risks, and certainly there are a lot of risks out there, more now than ever before. Fire fighting is a dangerous occupation. And it's just as dangerous for a volunteer. Fire knows no difference. Buildings that collapse know no difference. Someone who takes those risks and makes all the sacrifices without getting paid certainly needs to be admired.

Years ago the fire department strictly put out fires. But now that role has been expanded to many other areas, like car accidents and carbon monoxide testing. And the list goes on and on. There are also a lot of risks to helping people that weren't present years ago, like AIDS.

You have to be willing to take those risks and to make sacrifices. You're going to miss someone's birthday party; you're going to miss Christmas dinner, and you're going to miss your daughter's dance recital or basketball game. You'll miss a lot of those things. I know my family has made a lot of sacrifices over the years because things happen at inopportune times and you have to react.

Getting the Job Done

When there's a fire call, I think the first thing that happens is that your adrenaline takes over. I know myself—and I've been doing this for 23-plus years—that when your pager goes off, it startles you. It interrupts whatever you may be doing—even your full-time job. It often goes off when I'm at the prison, where I work as the assistant to the superintendent. And when it does, I might have to put my job on hold. Then you start to think a million things, "What is it? What's involved? What am I going to have to do?"

As a volunteer fire chief, I certainly look at it from a different perspective than I would have five or 10 years ago because my responsibilities were different. I might have been the officer who was taking a group of firefighters into a building. Now I'm responsible for all those firefighters and for coordinating the whole incident. And it's a monumental responsibility.

When you're working an incident, you rely on all the training that you've had over the years. Things just start to fall into place. A lot of it is very military-like, very structured. Although there may appear to be a lot of confusion, there are a lot of do's and don'ts that you follow from training. You just know what you're supposed to do.

For someone who has never gone inside a burning building, it's probably hard to imagine what it's like. It would be difficult enough if someone were to blindfold you and say, "I want you to walk around your office and find your way out." But we're going inside a building that's super-heated and smoky. We can't see our hands in front of our face. We're crawling on our hands and knees. To make matters worse, someone has just told us there's someone in there. Find them. At that point, we don't know if the roof is going to come down on us, if something is going to explode—or what the situation might be. But that's our job.

As fire chief, I can't say, "I don't know how to handle this, but I'll call somebody else who does." I can call for more help, but it's still my responsibility. I take my position as fire chief as seriously as a heart attack. I even went to school to earn a bachelor's degree in fire service administration. That's a credential most people in the fire service—even most full-time fire chiefs—don't have. But I look at it this way: Whatever time I have to put in, I put it in. My time's the investment, but I also want to see a result. I'm goal-oriented. I like to get things done. And I think because of all that, I've gained respect.

A Philosophy of Fairness

One of the people *I* respect is my father. Certainly over the years, we've had our differences, like any father and son. But I think some of the things he taught me at a young age, like the idea of being responsible, are very difficult to express to someone when they're age 14, 15, or 16—that what you're doing right now could come back to haunt you years down the road. Also, to tell the truth. A lot of those simple, basic things that at the time seem unimportant are values that stick with you throughout your life. The idea of being conservative and knowing the value of a dollar, not to spend frivolously, not to spend beyond your means—those are all things that I've done in my own life, and I now try to put into practice as chief of the fire department. You just don't whimsically go out and buy something that you can't afford. If there is a need, it has to be justified and plugged into a budget.

I have some other simple philosophies to live by. First of all, you have to trust people. You have to treat people the way you'd want to

be treated. You have to treat everyone fairly—then you don't have to worry about who you've treated unfairly.

I think the other thing is if you hold people accountable and responsible, then you'll get results. One of the things that I saw as a problem—and this is a typical thing that happens in a lot of organizations—is that the person who's the fire chief traditionally has been the person who does everything. You're the person who's obviously in charge at an emergency, but you're also the guy they call when something breaks, and you're the guy who's supposed to be there for every fund-raising event. In other words, you're the do-it-all because you're the fire chief. And that's not necessarily the case. You may be responsible, but you have to delegate your authority to other people. And if you do that, then they feel responsible and they'll get the job done. They'll also respect you because you treat them as more than just a token title.

I like to portray a positive image by being neat, clean, organized and well-prepared regardless of what I'm doing. I would not think of instructing a fire training program without being spit and polished and dressing the part. I think all of that is an image thing. That's not to say that I don't let my hair down at times. But that's how you gain respect. People have a certain expectation of how a fire chief should look. And my kids have an expectation of what their father should look like and how he should behave. It would be very difficult to preach to them and then have them or someone else see me stagger out of a barroom or out of my house. So I practice what I preach.

Living and working by these simple philosophies has brought me both respect and success. There are not a whole lot of things I've failed at. There *are* a lot of things I probably would have done a little bit differently, but there's nothing I would say I tried and I fell flat on my face. Anything I may have failed at, I look at as just a temporary inconvenience that has made me stronger and a better person.

Taking the Path Less Traveled

Trevor Murphy, Moshi, Tanzania, East Africa

Date of birth: August 4, 1972

Profession: Peace Corps volunteer

When I graduated from the University of California at Berkeley in 1994 with a degree in economics, I wasn't sure what I wanted to do. I tried the path most graduates with an economics degree take—I got a job with an investment banking firm. But after about six months of working 10- to 12-hour days, in an office, at a desk, and wearing a suit and tie, the money just wasn't worth it. So I decided to apply to the Peace Corps.

I had never done volunteer work before, at least not anything beyond my once-a-year commitment to the Special Olympics. I never had time between working so I could financially stay in school, and studying so I could academically stay in school. But there I was, a recent graduate of college, I wasn't enjoying my first taste of the working world, and I had always been intrigued with other cultures. I figured a two-year stint in another country wasn't that long, and I had the rest of my life to work at a desk.

A few months after I applied, I got a phone call from the Peace Corps asking me if I wanted to go to East Africa to teach economics. I made one of those instant decisions over the phone and said yes before I knew what I was saying. It was probably one of the best decisions I've made in my life.

Scaling the Heights

I never thought I would be a teacher. But here I am teaching at Weruweru, an all-female boarding school located in Moshi, Tanzania.

Weruweru is an advanced-level, or A-level, school for students between the ages of 16 and 21. My students had to take a national examination in their subjects to study at this advanced level. (Only a small percentage of students who begin school actually make it to the A level, so my students are exceptional students by Tanzanian standards.)

Even though my students are exceptional academically, teaching has been very challenging. There is the language barrier—I teach in English, and they are still learning the English language. And there is the cultural barrier—Tanzania is a patriarchal society, and the traditional roles for women are very rigid. Women are expected to get married, have children, and stay at home to support the family and the farm. Tanzanian women don't have a lot of confidence in themselves and understanding of the options that are available to them. I am constantly trying to encourage my students to keep working at their studies to try to break out of this traditional mold. And it has been very rewarding to see my students succeed.

The town of Moshi is located at the base of Mount Kilimanjaro—the highest point in Africa (19,341 feet). Kilimanjaro is a volcano that towers over my school, and its immensity beckons you to climb.

Despite the fact that I had never climbed before, after a few weeks in Moshi, I was beckoned. And for purely selfish reasons—I was determined to make the climb up Kilimanjaro—I decided to make it an educational trip and take some of my students. I figured that with the support of Weruweru, I could make it to the top much quicker...that is, if my students would make the trek.

I announced at morning assembly that I would be climbing Kilimanjaro, and whoever was interested in joining me should meet in my classroom after school. I didn't think anyone would show up. The thought of climbing Kilimanjaro had probably never entered my students' minds. They are women, and as far as they were concerned, Kilimanjaro is reserved for strong men and wealthy tourists. But to my delight, a number of women came ready to train.

I started a rigorous program so that only those who were really hungry for the challenge would continue to train. We had seven weeks to get ready, and we began meeting after school to run and do calisthenics. It was challenging because exercise is not something these women had ever done before, at least not on purpose.

The Few, The Proud

From the beginning, no one believed that young African women would make it to the top—I had a hard time convincing my students as well. But I think the negative talk just made them work even harder to prove those people wrong. As the training progressed, and the day of the climb approached, I began to grasp how important this hike would be for my students. The climb had become less about me and my personal goals to see the summit, and more about my students and their determination to prove themselves.

Kilimanjaro is a six-day climb that isn't technically difficult—there's a path that leads the way up the mountain—but it is a steep climb on a trail that is covered with shale. So, for each step forward, you slide half a step back. And it is slow-moving. You have to take your time on the climb so your body can adjust to new altitudes. There isn't enough oxygen up there for heavy breathing.

At the time that we reached the summit, I was tired and wrapped up in making sure that all my students were okay—some of them were scattered behind us on the trail, keeled over with altitude sickness. I didn't have an opportunity to relax until we were all safely back down the hill. After all the dust cleared, and we were all together again, I felt really proud. Proud that I made it, but even prouder that my students made it. Seeing the expressions on their faces when we reached the summit was one of the best experiences of my life. It was a beautiful, unforgettable moment.

On Top of the World

Since we completed the hike, we have had a flood of positive attention from the media and political figures. When First Lady Hillary Rodham Clinton and her daughter, Chelsea, were in Tanzania for a visit, my students were invited to a roundtable discussion with the Clintons and several Tanzanian officials. Nine of my students who had made it to the summit performed a poem they had written about climbing Kilimanjaro. It was very emotional.

More important, my students have an air of confidence that wasn't there before. For us, the climb was a challenge to build our inner selves. But because this was a first for African women, it has come to represent something larger. It has been a positive step for all African women in their struggle to prove their strength and break down traditional barriers.

The confidence my students gained has influenced them academically. I'm proud to say that some of my students recently passed the TOEFL (Teaching of English as a Foreign Language) exam that tests a student's mastery of English for university study abroad. Now I just have to help them find some scholarships. I feel great satisfaction in knowing that I was a part of this positive change in their lives.

I have decided to extend my time with the Peace Corps by an additional six months so I can finish the academic year with my students. Afterward, I think I would like to come back to Tanzania on a Fulbright Scholarship to help set up career resource centers and TOEFL centers so students can see their options, be they continuing education or working somewhere other than the family farm.

Through all my Tanzanian adventures, I have learned one truth: When you try to get your students high on a mountain, you can find yourself close to the summit as well.

Index